A NICU Book for the Whole Family!

Table of Contents

AF208066

Parenting Tips for Supporting Your Children
During a NICU Stay **3**

Our New Baby in the NICU **5**
(A book for young children
and children with short attention spans.)

Drawing Activity for Families.. **23**

All About Our Baby and the NICU................................. **25**
(A book with more NICU explanations
and details for kids who like to know more.)

Discussion Questions for the Whole Family............... **49**

We Love You Everywhere and All of the Time............. **51**
(A book for parents and older kids
to read to their new baby.)

Dedicated to all of the women and men who give so much themselves to take care of these sweet babies and their families. I have learned so much from so many of you.

A special thank you to the NICU staff that helped edit and advise.

This first two books are intended to be read to a child by a trusted adult.

The advice and words within this book may not be suitable for every child or every situation. In especially stressful or complex situations, this author suggests the involvement of a mental health profesional.

The last book in this collection is meant to be read to a baby. Please monitor for any signs of stress while reading and stop reading if baby shows any signs of distress.

ISBN Paperback 978-1-7367884-5-5

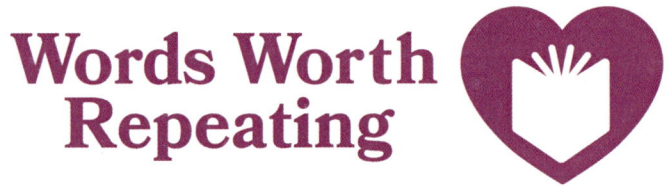

www.wordsworthrepeating.com

Tips for Supporting a Sibling during a NICU Stay

-Ask staff if your NICU has a Child Life Specialist. Consult this hospital professional for free advice and support for the baby's sibling.

 -If allowed and appropriate, bring the big brother or sister to visit the baby in the NICU. Prepare the brother or sister before they go into the NICU. Reading this book and talking about what they will see is one way to prepare a child. The first time the child visits, it is important to have another adult with you. This will give you some flexibility, if your child is ready to go, and you need to stay.

 -For younger children, have a baby doll at home that allows your child to play through what they are experiencing. When you have time, consider playing "hospital" with your child. Play is how children learn.

 -Take a photo of the big brother or sister to the NICU and attach it to the baby's crib. Show the big brother/sister a picture of their new baby next to the photo.

 -Don't make any promises. Babies and healthcare are hard to predict. Even if a nurse or doctor tells you that you will probably "go home tomorrow", prepare your child with "our baby MIGHT come home tomorrow". Babies can have a spell, lowered heart rate, or lab result that keeps them in the NICU for a few more days.

NICU Parents,

This book is for you, too! The NICU is full of medical jargon and sleepless nights that can make parents' brains foggy. As adults, sometimes we need things to be simple. May these short explanations help you revisit complicated issues in a simple way and feel good about the ways you are supporting all of your children.

Not being able to be with your children all the time is SO hard. Always remember, kids are incredibly resilient! Your family will get through this. In the mean time, here is a little advice that I've gotten from years of working with NICU parents:

-If people offer help, take it or tell them what would be even more helpful.

-Take care of you. When this baby comes home, he/she is going to need all of you. Get rest, eat good food, and give yourself time to heal (physically and mentally)!

-Lastly, remember that in the NICU, you are an advocate for you and for your baby. Trust your gut. If you notice a change or something seems off, say something. Talk to these strangers who are now taking care of one of your baby... many will become friends. Be open with them. When they understand where you are coming from, they can better care for you and your baby. Ask questions until you understand or ask them to expain it in another way. You are this new little human's voice and most important caretaker. Don't feel silly for asking for more information. If anything, they should feel silly for not explaining it in a better way.

You've got this!

Laura

Our New Baby in the NICU

Book 1: Short and Simple

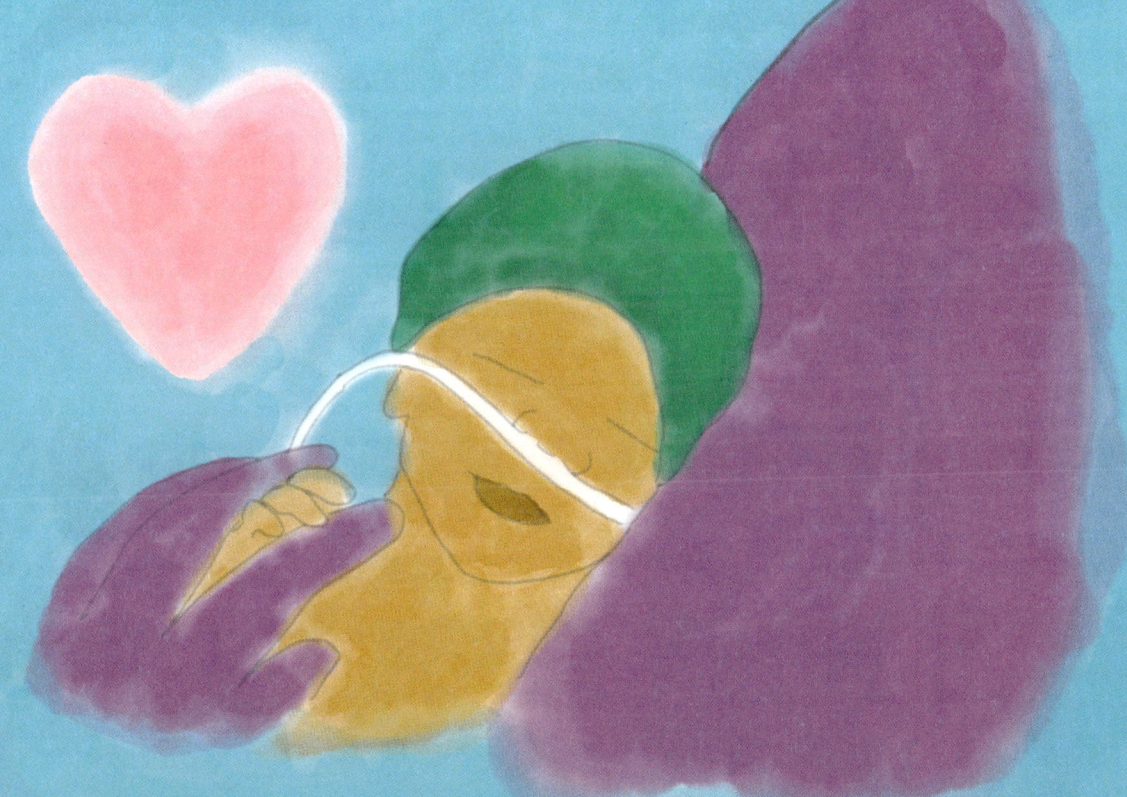

Written and Illustrated by Laura Camerona, CCLS

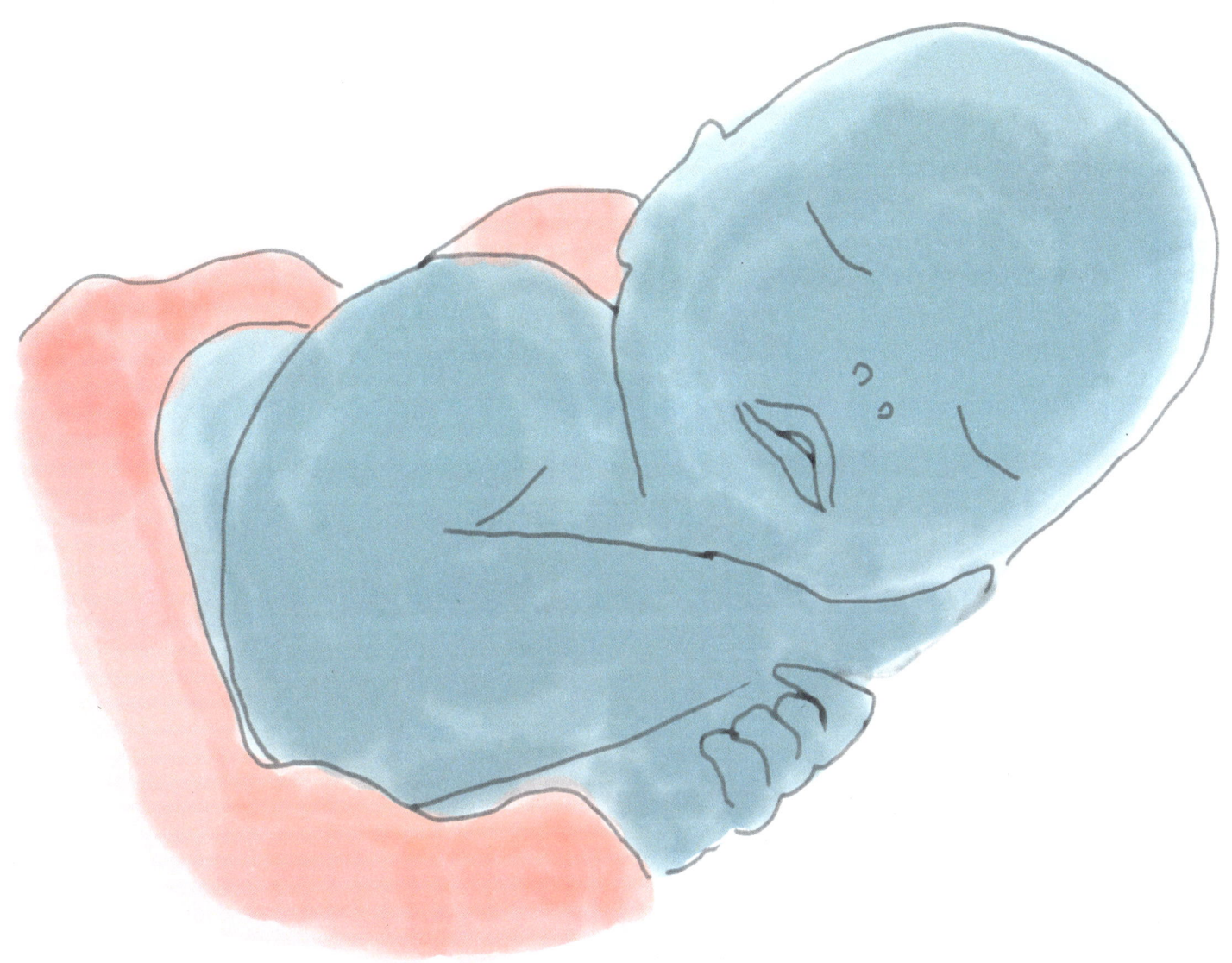

There is a new baby in our family. Our new baby's name is
Bennett_____. I am the baby's new big
sister!_____ (brother/sister)!

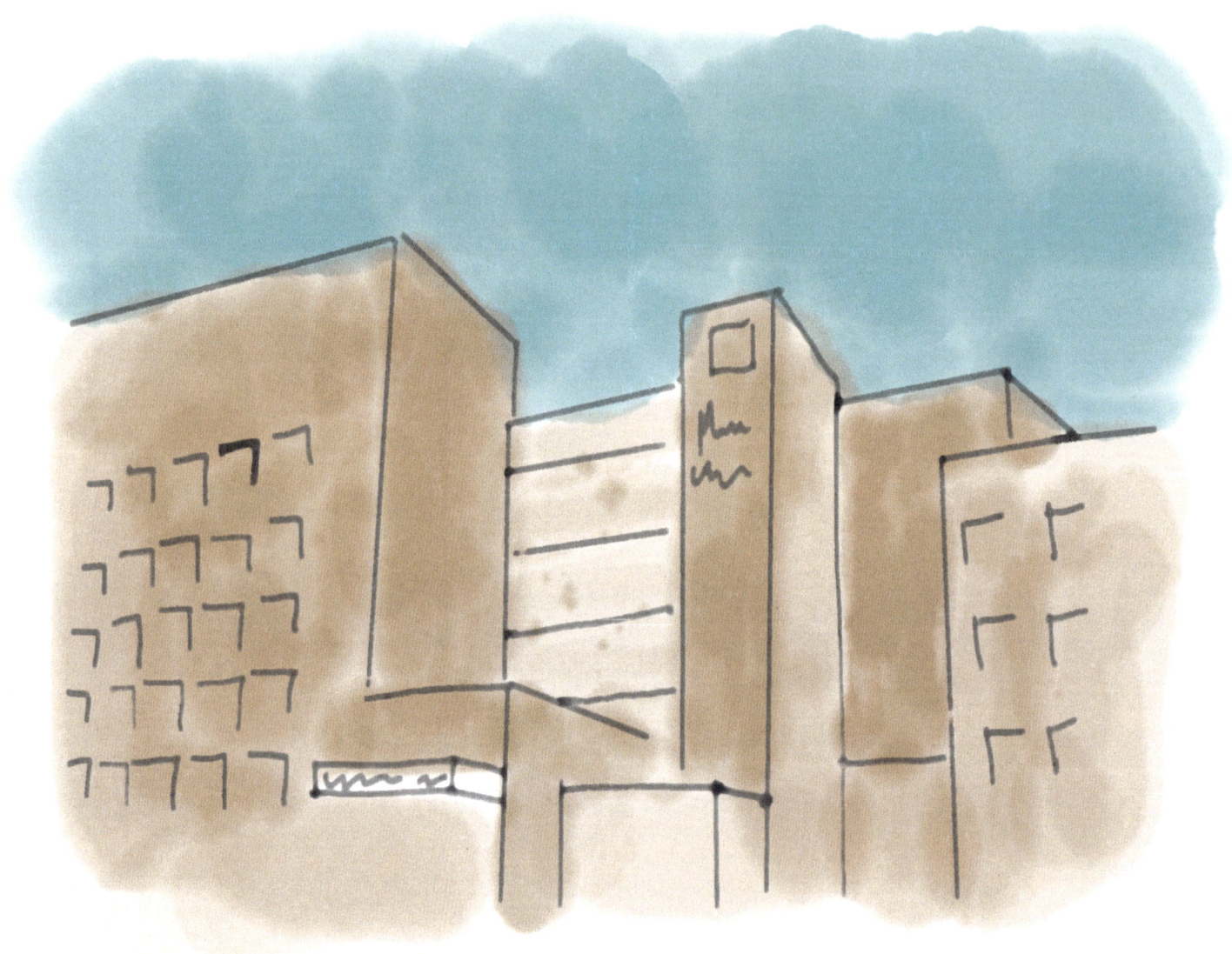

Right now, our new baby has to stay at the hospital. Our baby is in a special part of the hospital called the NICU.

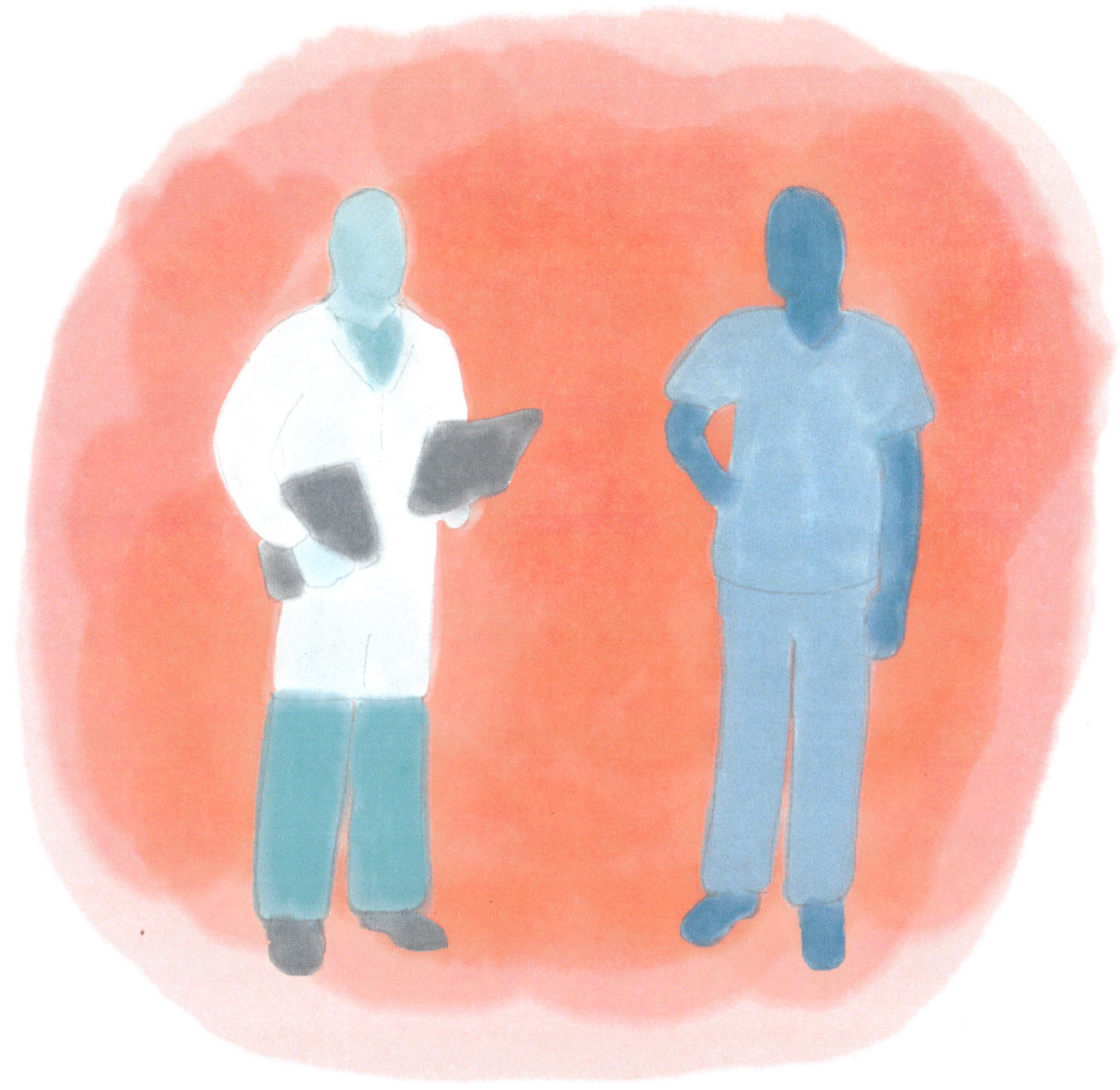

The doctors, nurses, and other people who work in the NICU have taken care of a lot of babies. They will take very good care of our baby!

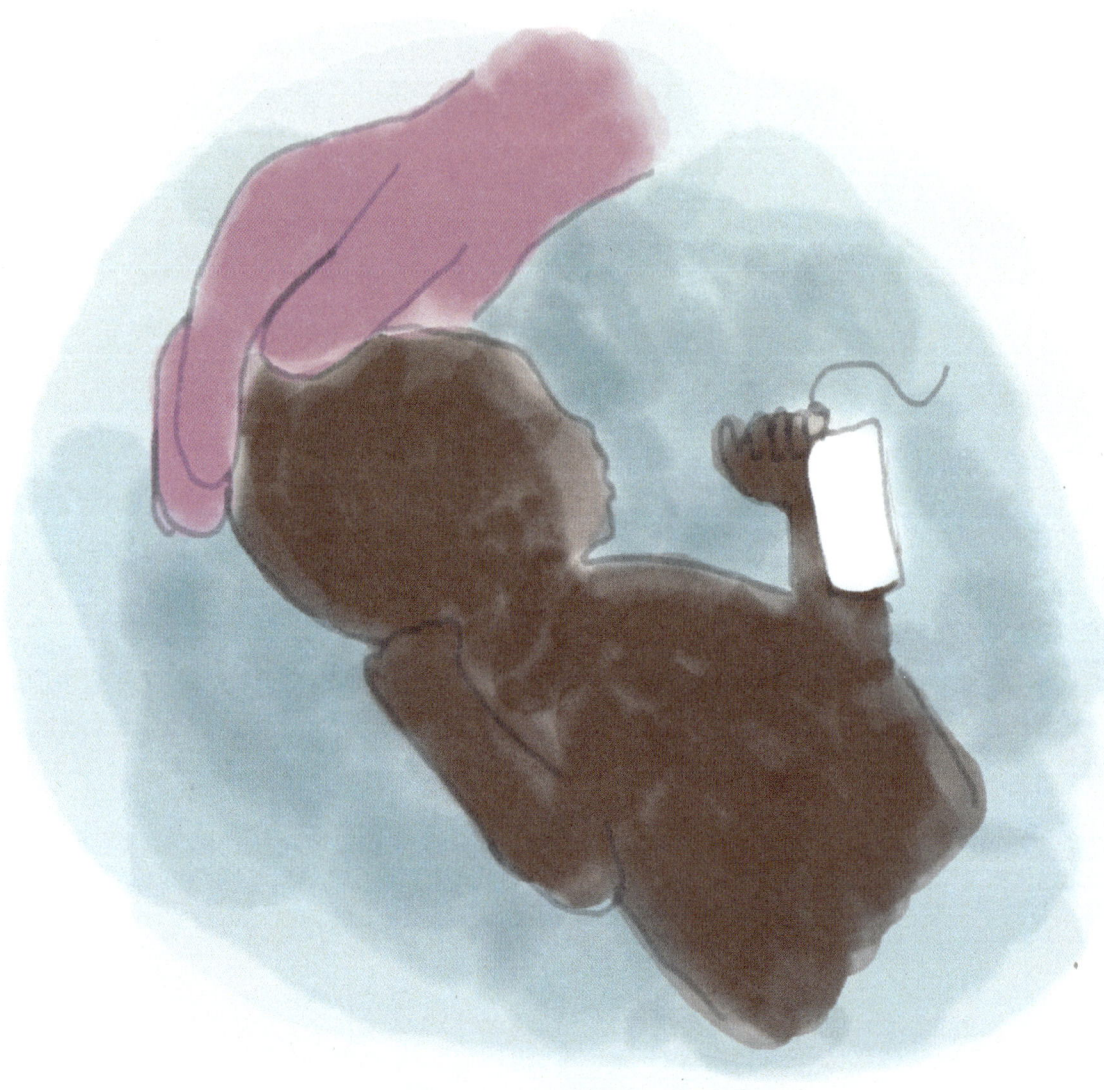

Our baby is not the only baby in the NICU. Babies that need extra help before they are ready to go home stay in the NICU.

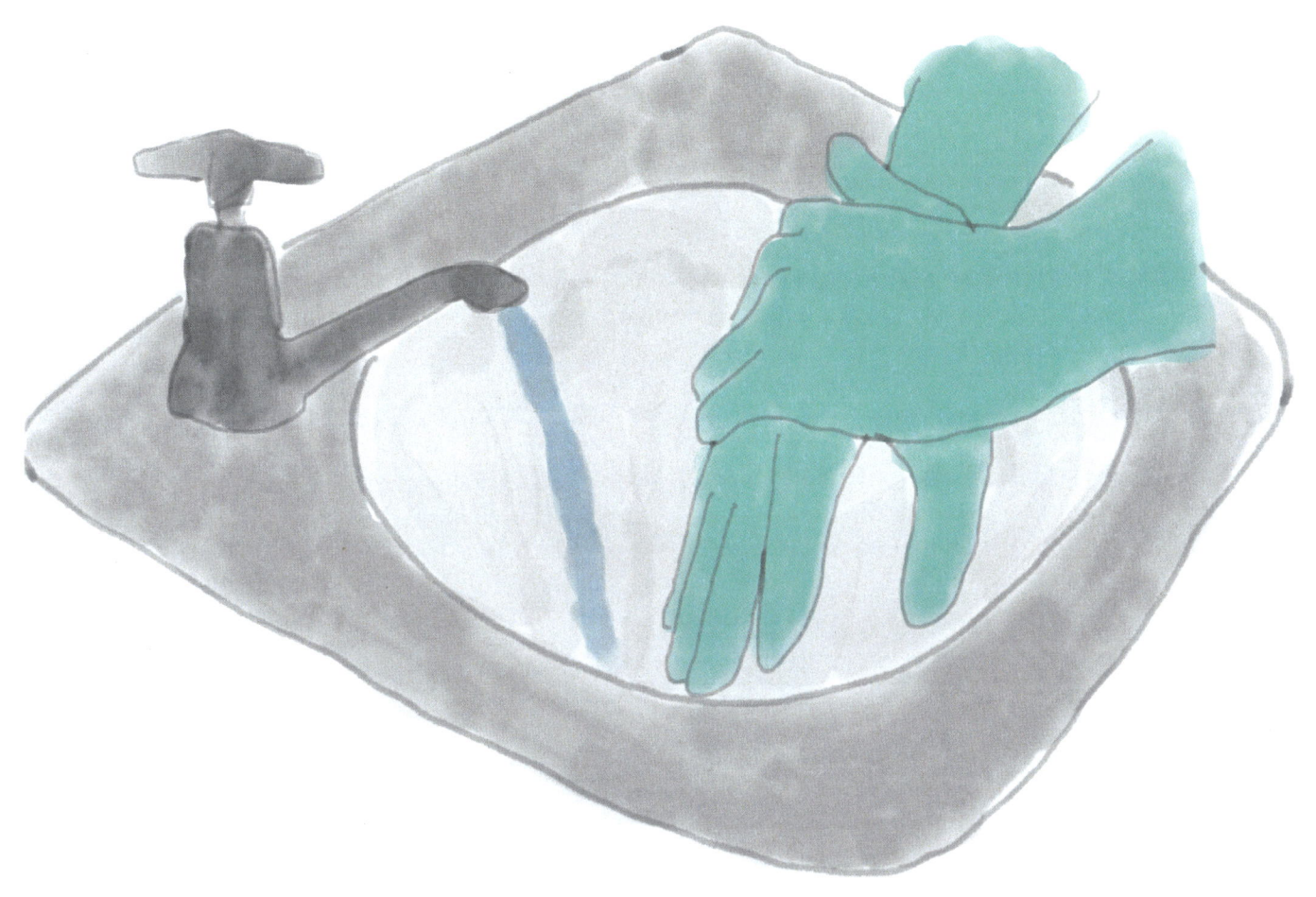

It is important to keep germs away from the babies in the NICU. Everyone in the NICU washes their hands a lot. People can not visit the NICU if they are sick.

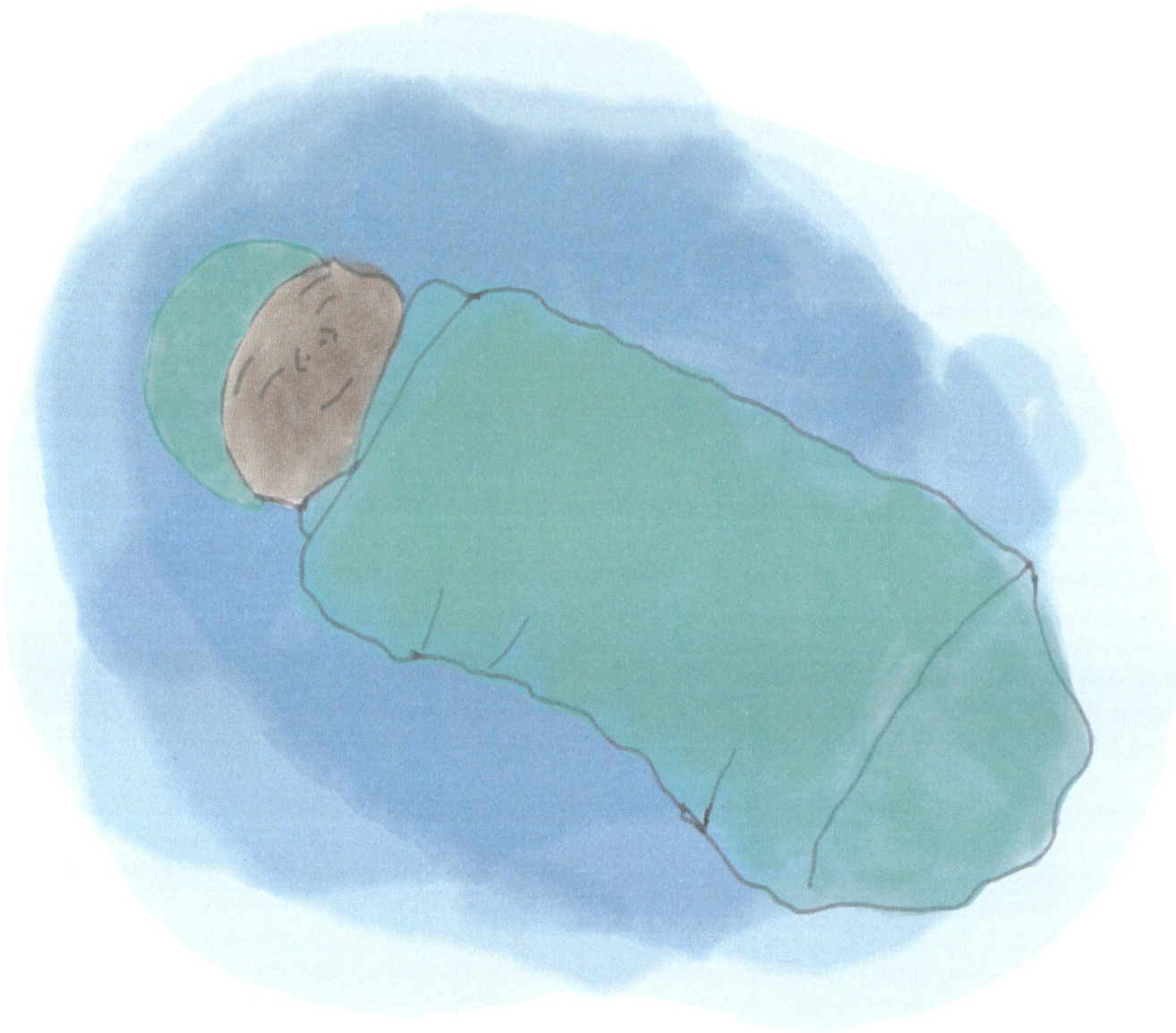

New babies need lots of rest to help their bodies grow big and strong. Everyone in the NICU needs to use quiet voices so that the babies can rest.

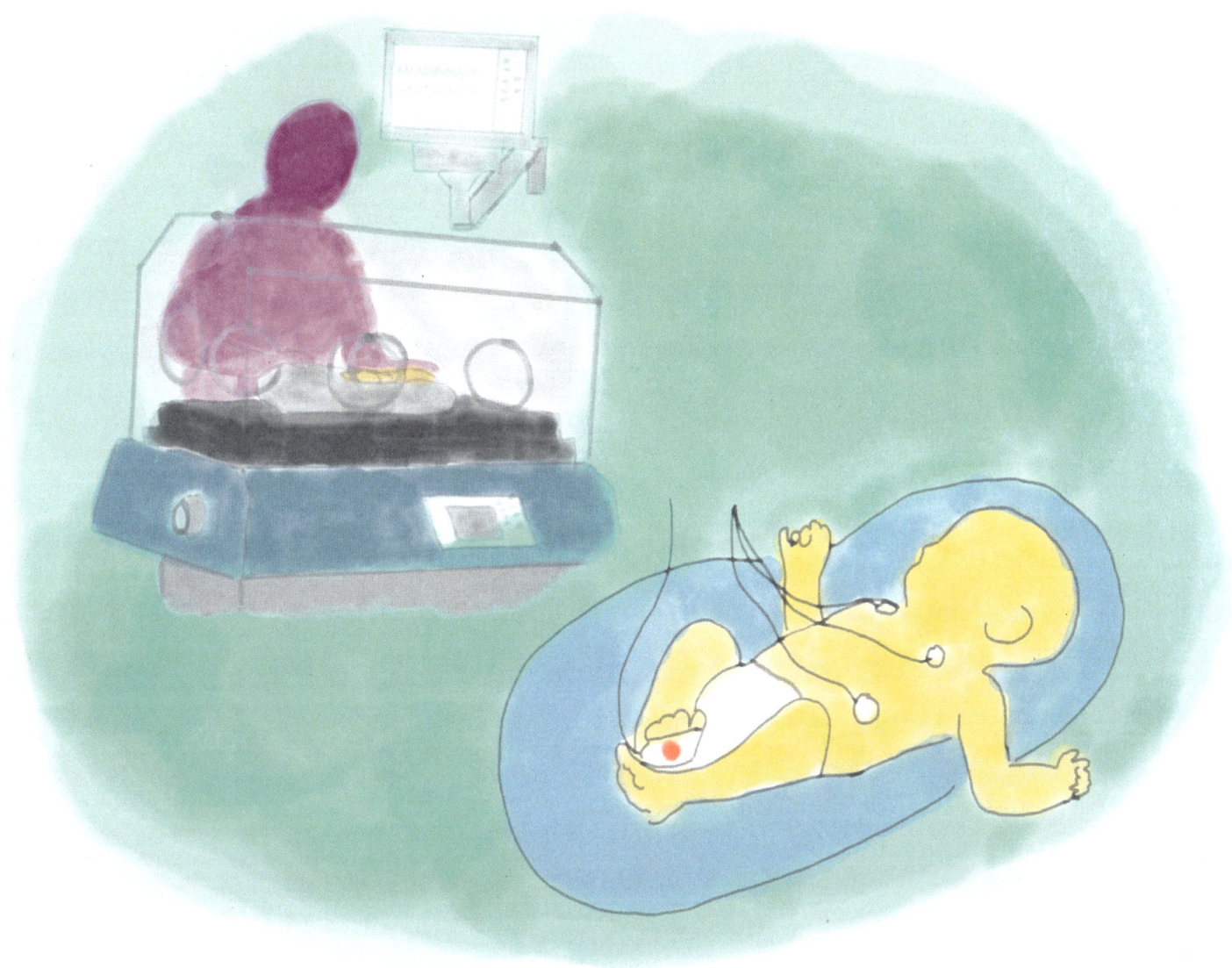

The doctors and nurses watch the babies carefully. Each baby wears a small red light on his or her foot and stickers on his or her chest that measure the baby's breathing and heartbeat. The doctors and nurses can see the measurements on a computer screen.

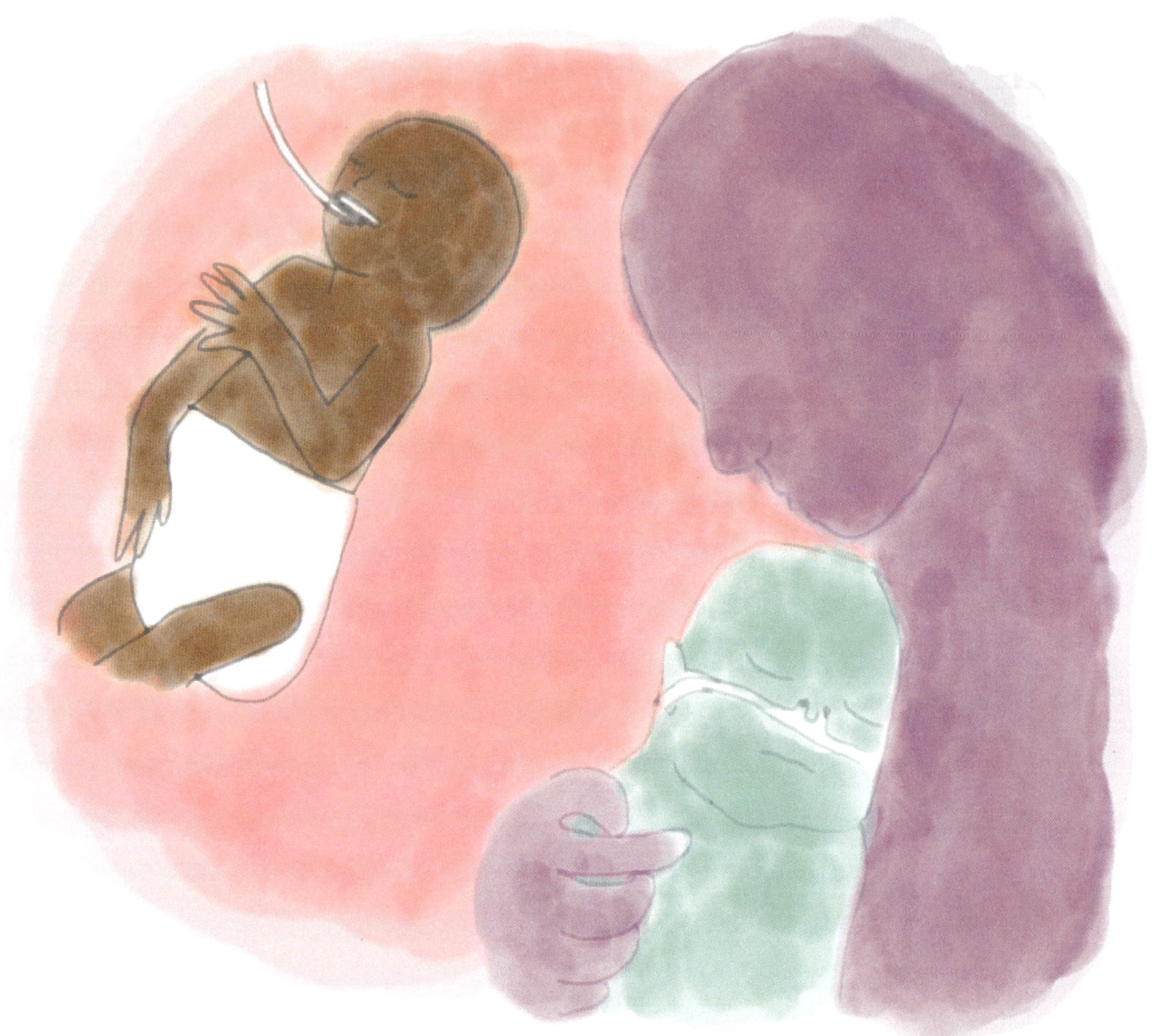

A baby that needs help breathing may have an oxygen tube that rests by his or her nose. If a baby needs more help, the baby may have a breathing tube in his or her mouth. The tube is connected to a machine that breathes for the baby called a ventilator.

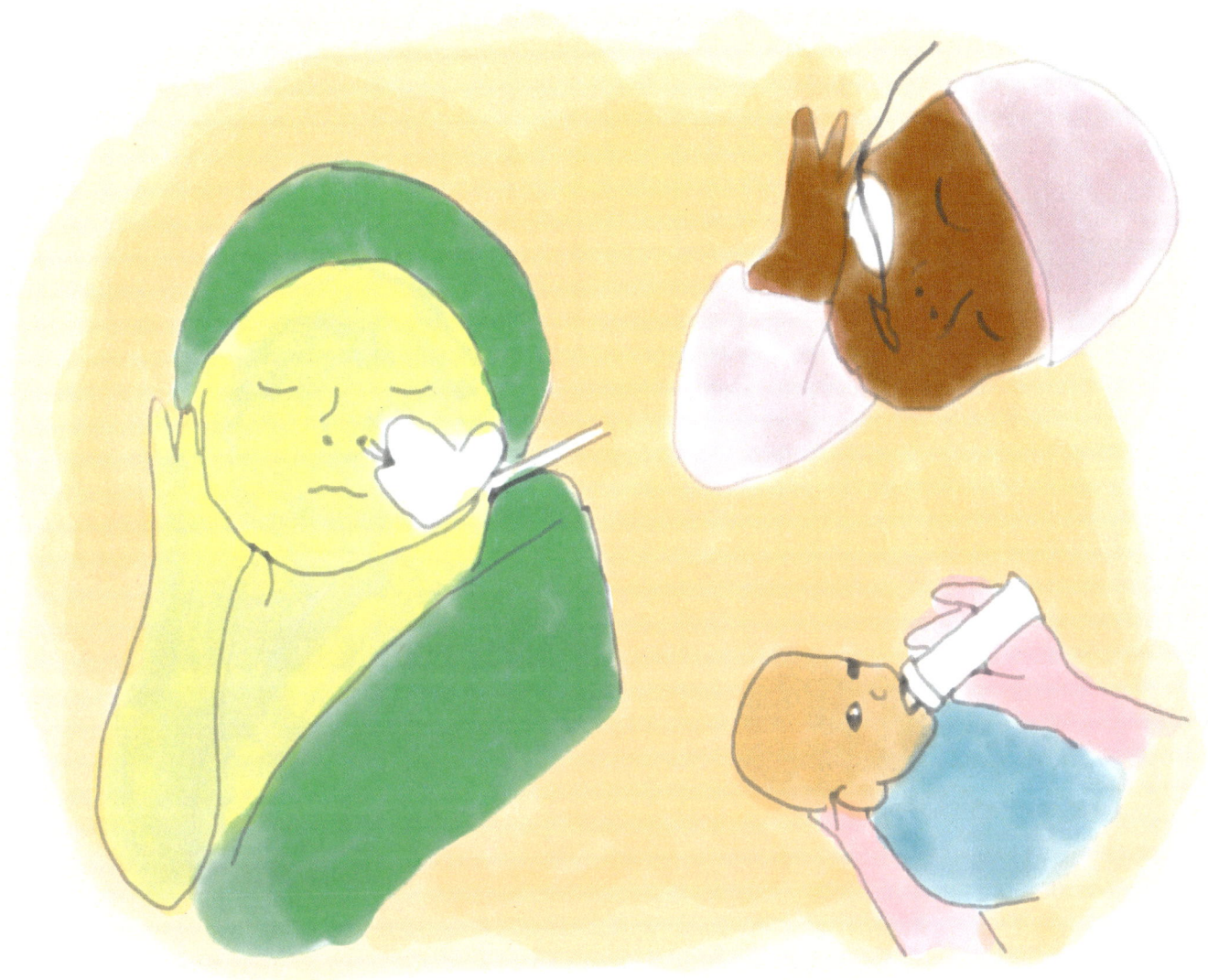

Some babies need help learning how to drink milk. If a baby does not drink all of its milk, a nurse can put the rest of the milk in a tiny feeding tube. Feeding tubes go in the baby's nose or mouth and help the milk get to the baby's tummy.

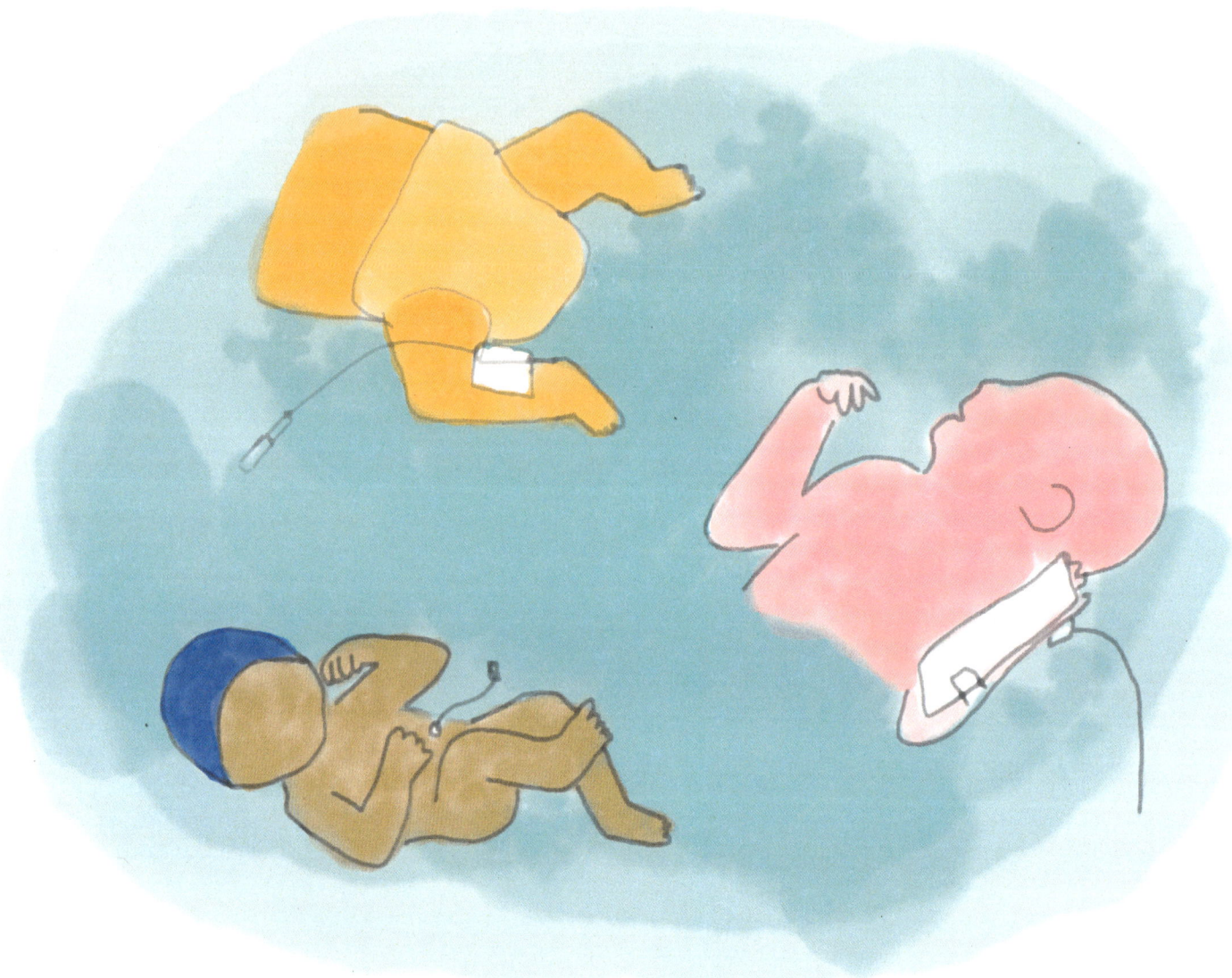

Babies may also have another tube called an IV. The nurses can use an IV to give the baby medicine. An IV can be on a baby's hand, foot, belly button, or head. IVs help the babies get all the medicine that they need.

Babies tell us that they need something by crying. A baby may cry because he or she is tired, hungry, or if something doesn't feel good. If a baby is crying, a nurse, doctor, or parent will check on the baby and help them.

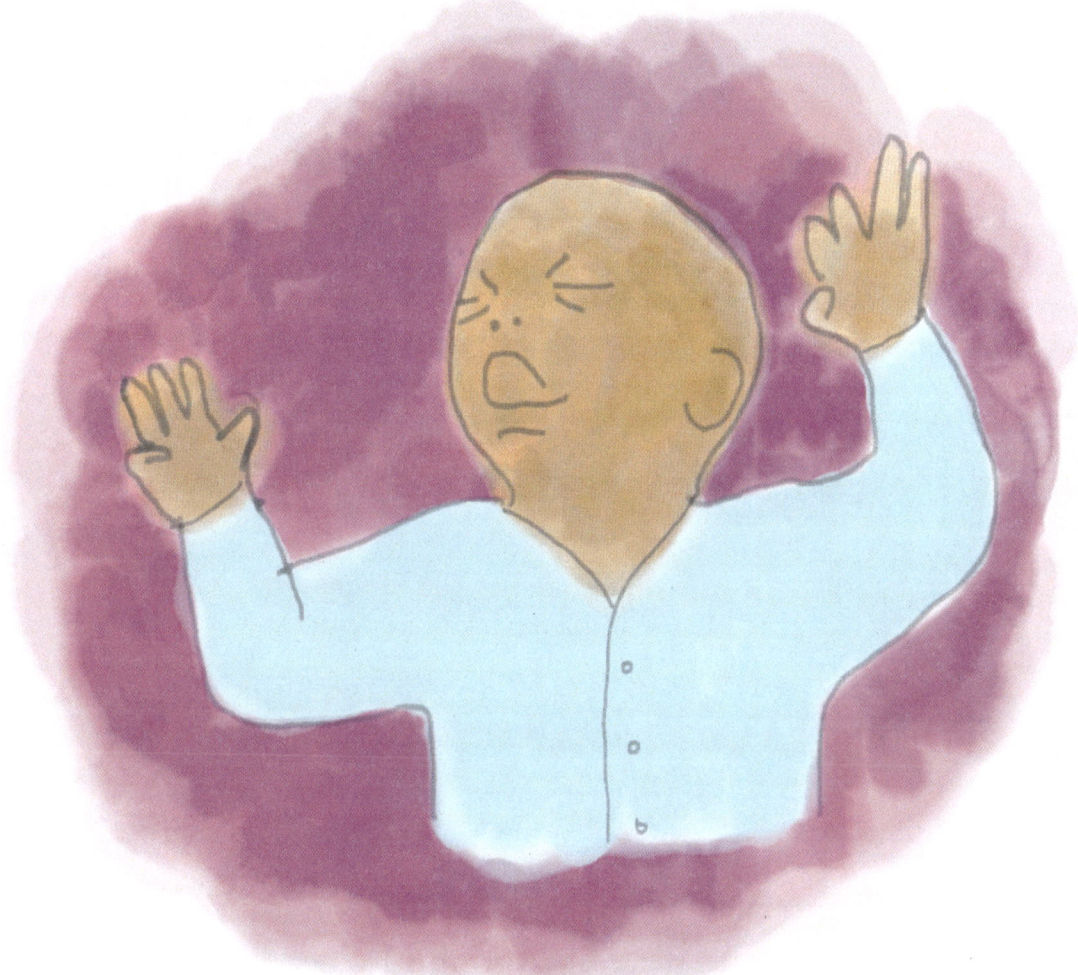

When our baby comes home, our parent will check on the baby when it cries. Crying is okay, but if I don't like it, I can find a quiet place to go and take a break.

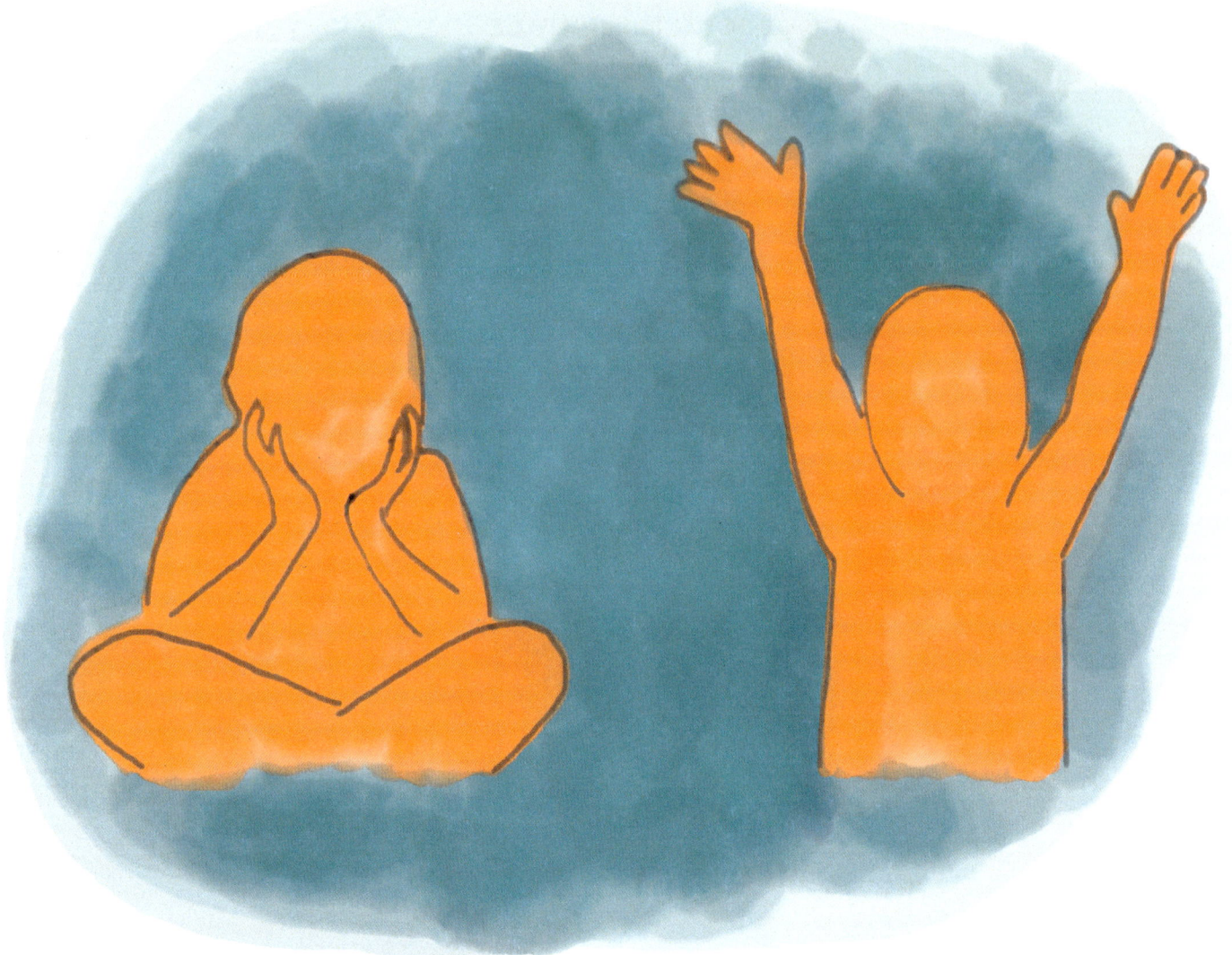

Being a new brother or sister, I might have lots of new feelings. I might feel happy that the new baby is finally here. I might feel sad that the baby has to stay at the hospital. Sometimes, I might feel jealous that people are focused on the baby and not me. All of those feelings are okay. I can talk to my family about them.

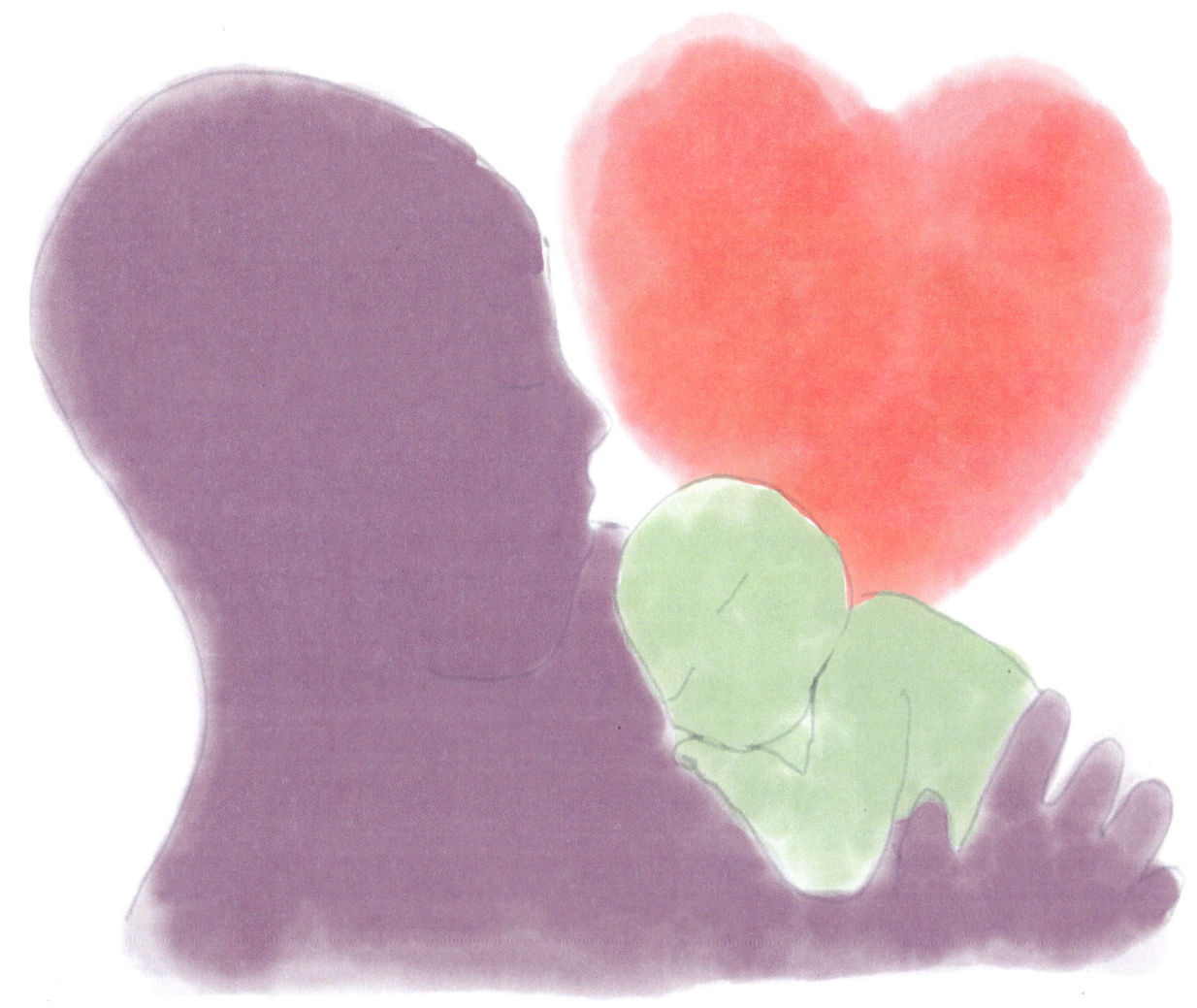

I miss my parent when they are at the hospital taking care of our baby, but when they are there, they are doing a very important job. My parent loves me and our new baby. I know when my parent isn't with me they still love me SO MUCH!

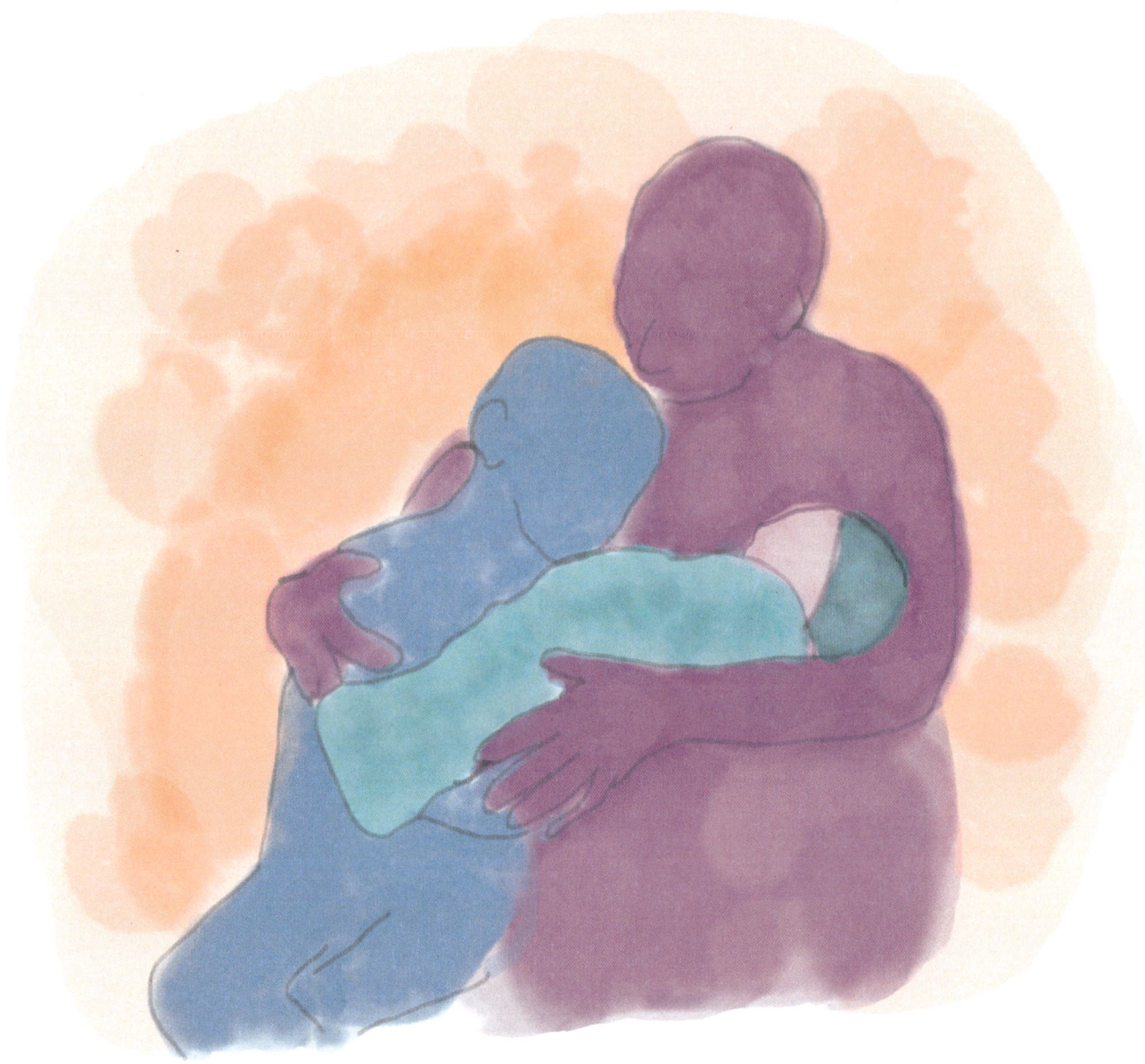

It will feel so good to have my whole family home together. Our baby will be able to come home when our baby is healthy and can drink enough milk to keep growing bigger and stronger. I can't wait for our baby to come home!

20

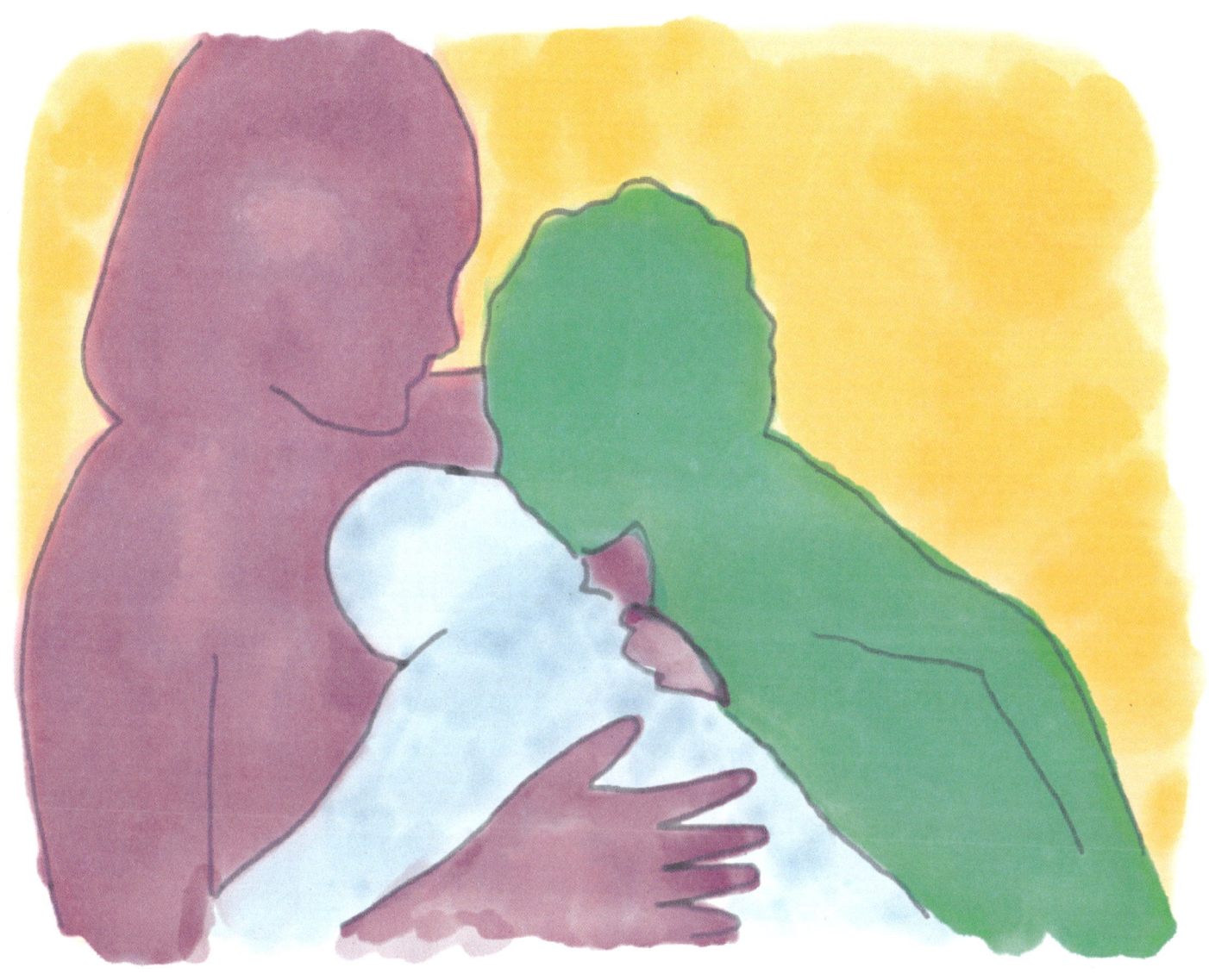

When our baby is home, my parent can help me hold our baby. I can help get diapers for the baby and sing to the baby.

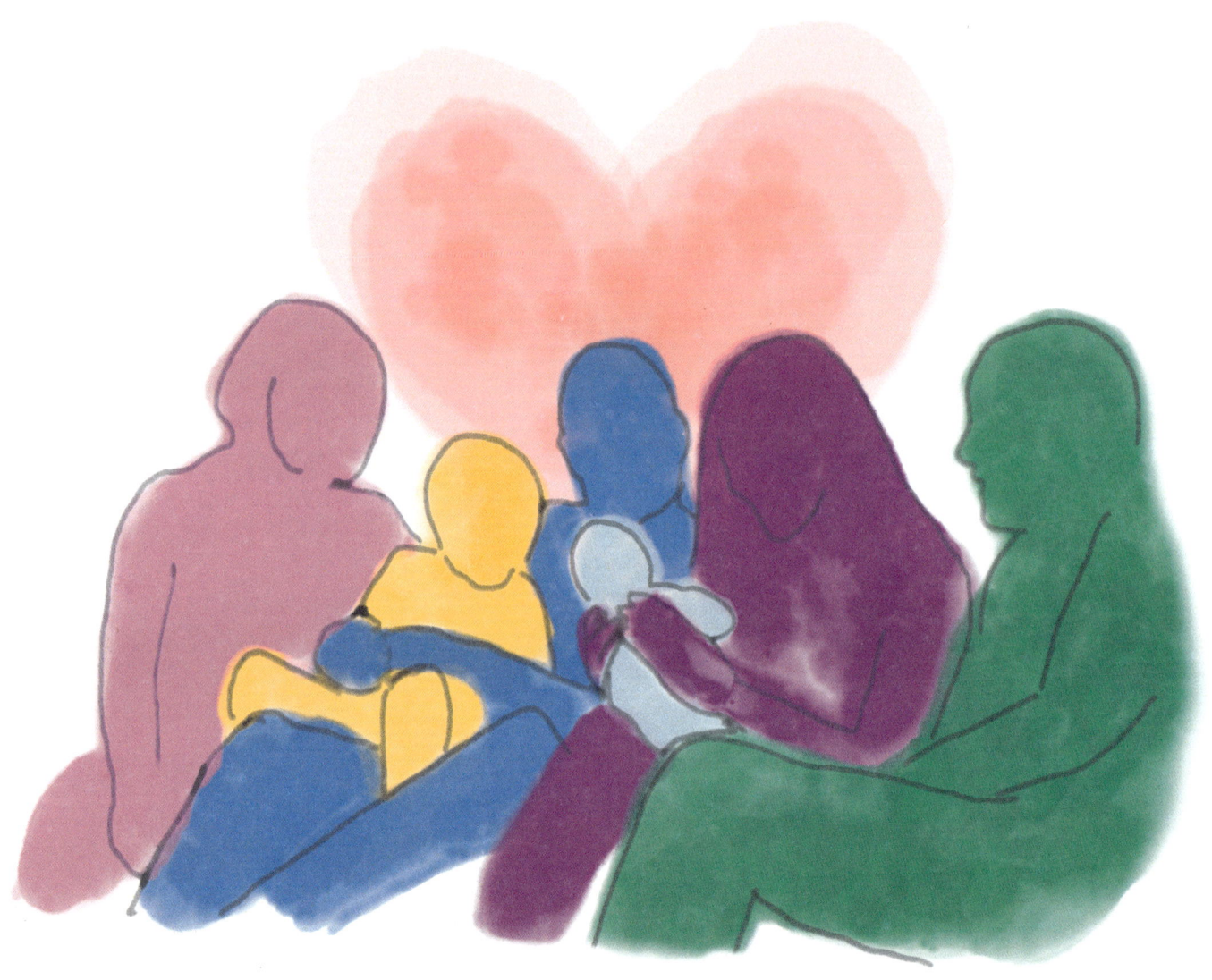

I am part of a big team of people who care about our baby! I am a great big _____(brother/sister)!

My picture of our new baby in the NICU.
(Drawing a picture with crayon or colored pencil is a great job for a
new brother or sister! Someday, your baby will love seeing it!)

My picture of our whole family together!

All About Our Baby and the NICU

Book 2: For Those Who Want to Know More

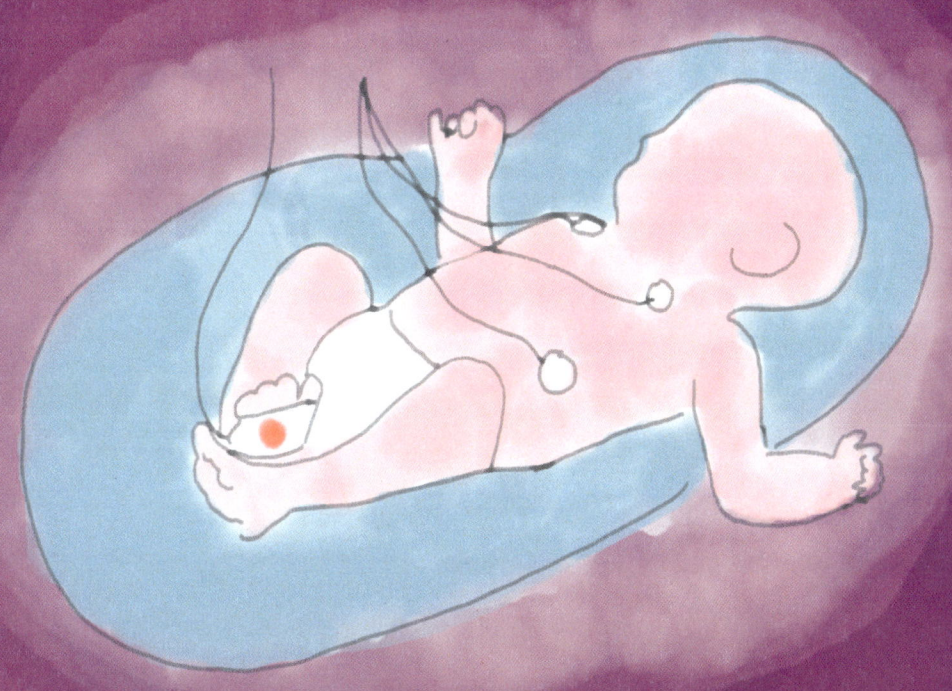

Written and Illustrated by
Laura Camerona, CCLS

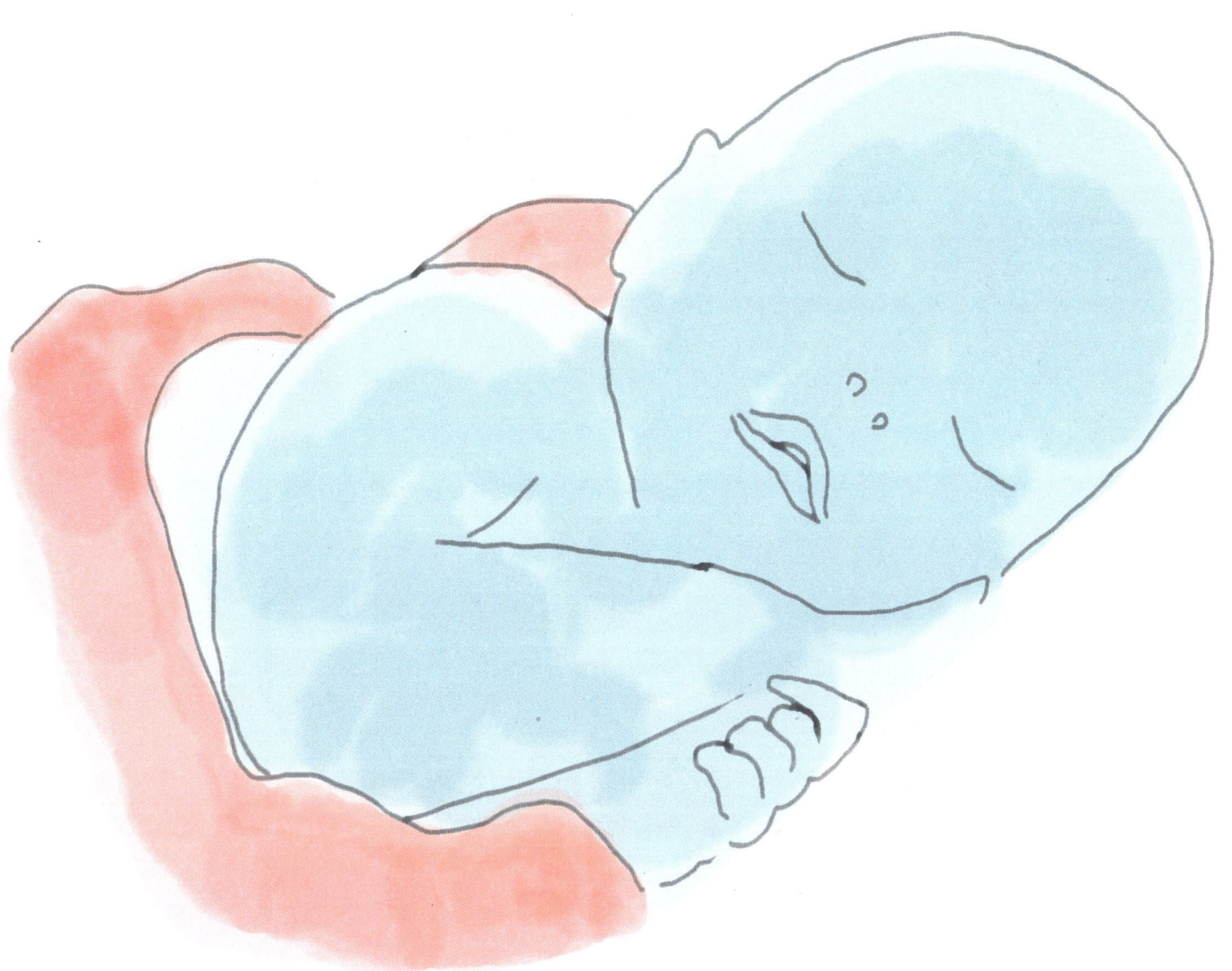

There is a new baby in our family. Our baby is named
_____.

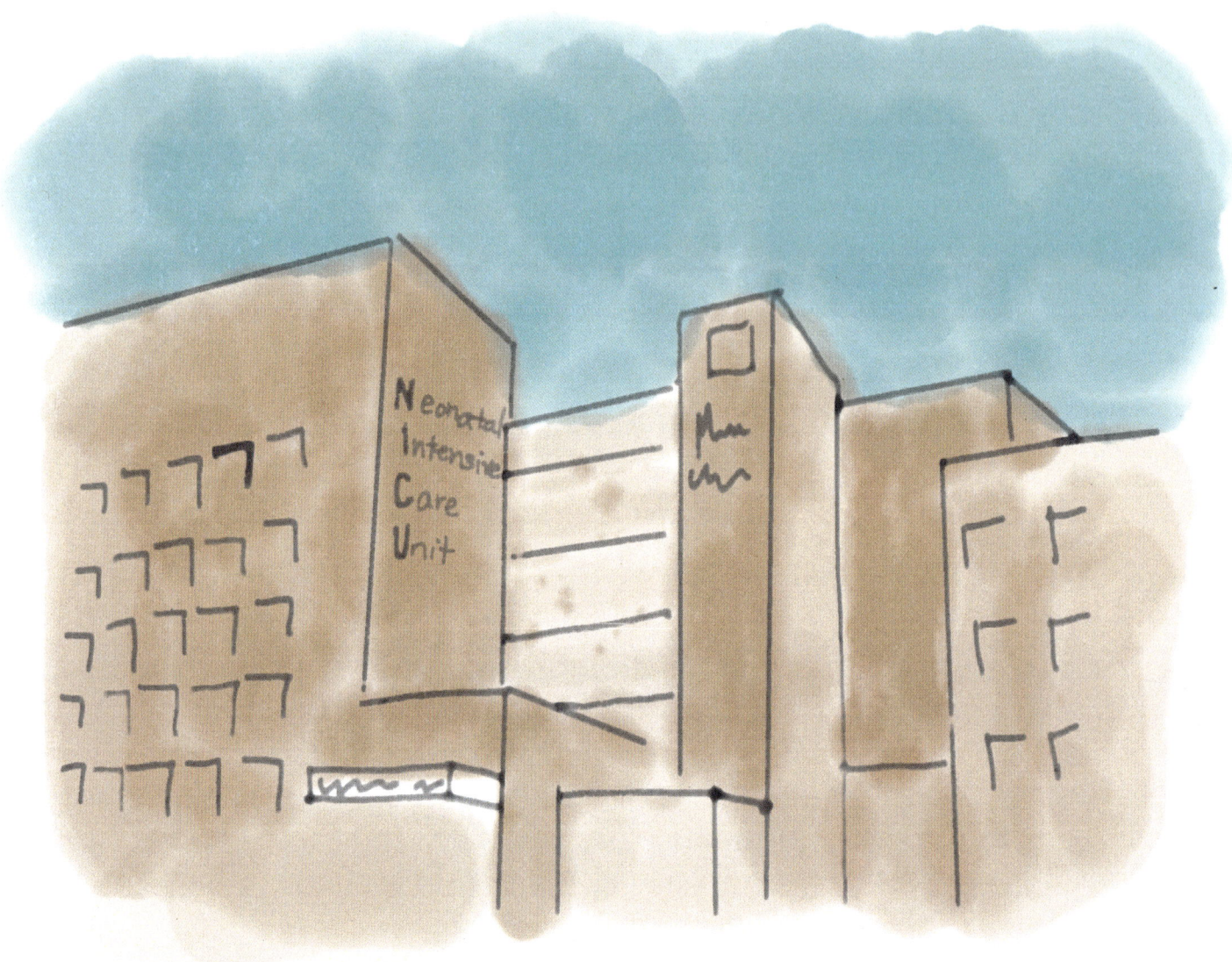

Right now, our new baby has to stay at the hospital. Our baby is in a special part of the hospital called the NICU. The NICU is where babies stay when they need to work on getting healthy or getting bigger before they can go home.

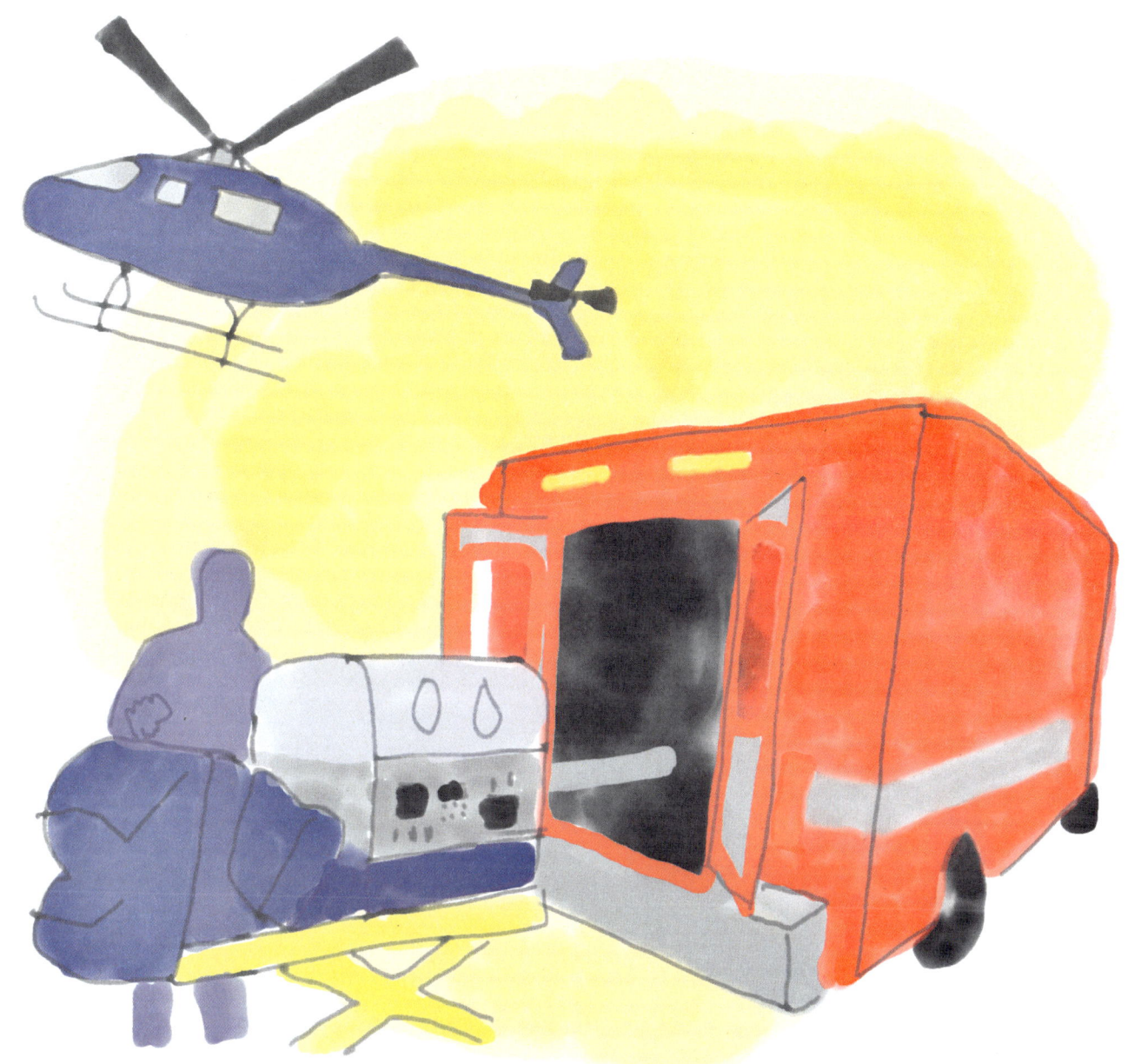

Some babies are born in the same hospital as the NICU. Other babies have to be brought to the NICU from another hospital. These babies can ride in an ambulance or in a helicopter.

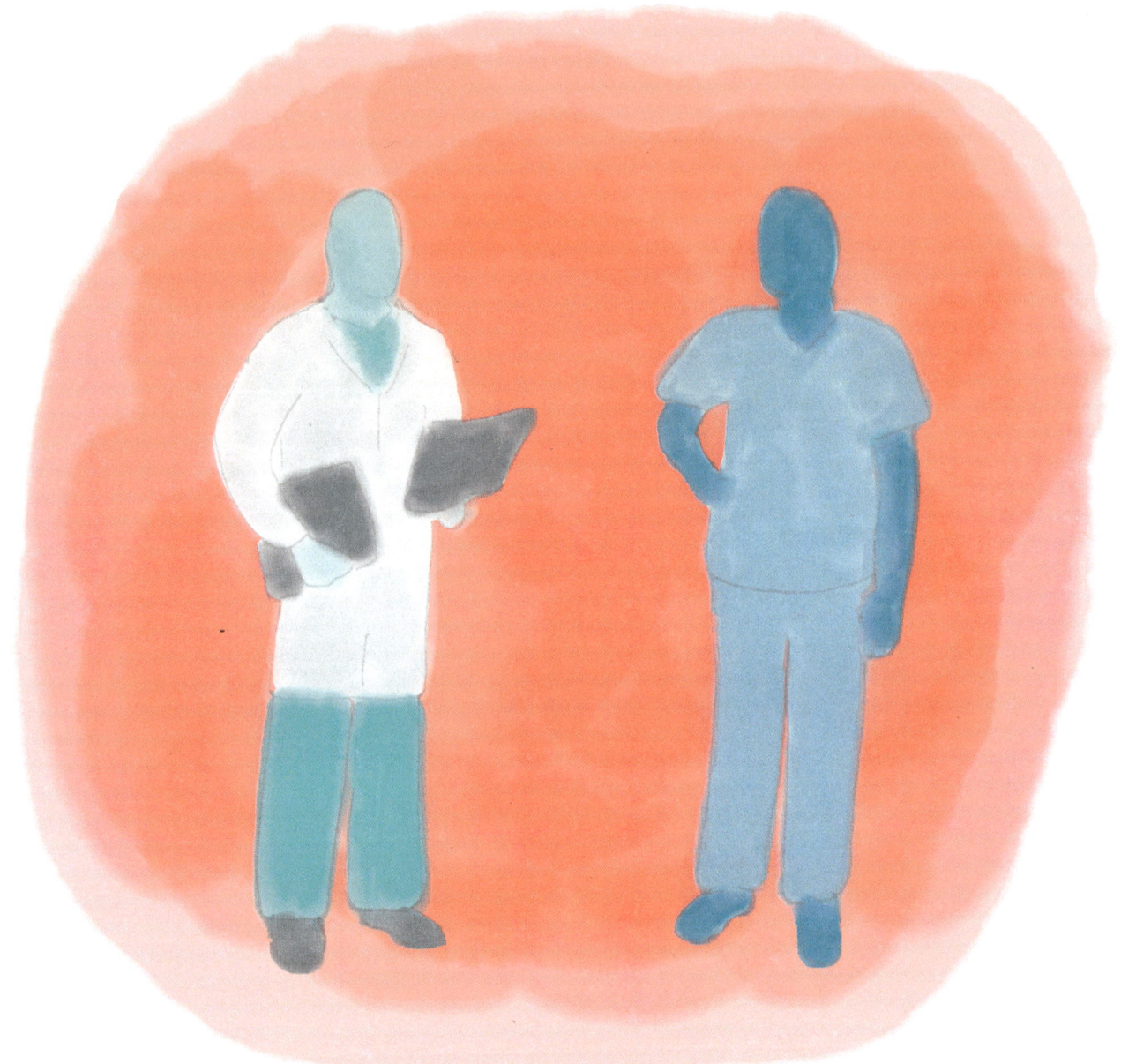

The NICU has nurses and doctors that take very good care of babies. They pay very close attention to our new baby. Many of them have taken care of babies for a long time and know a lot about how to help babies get healthy.

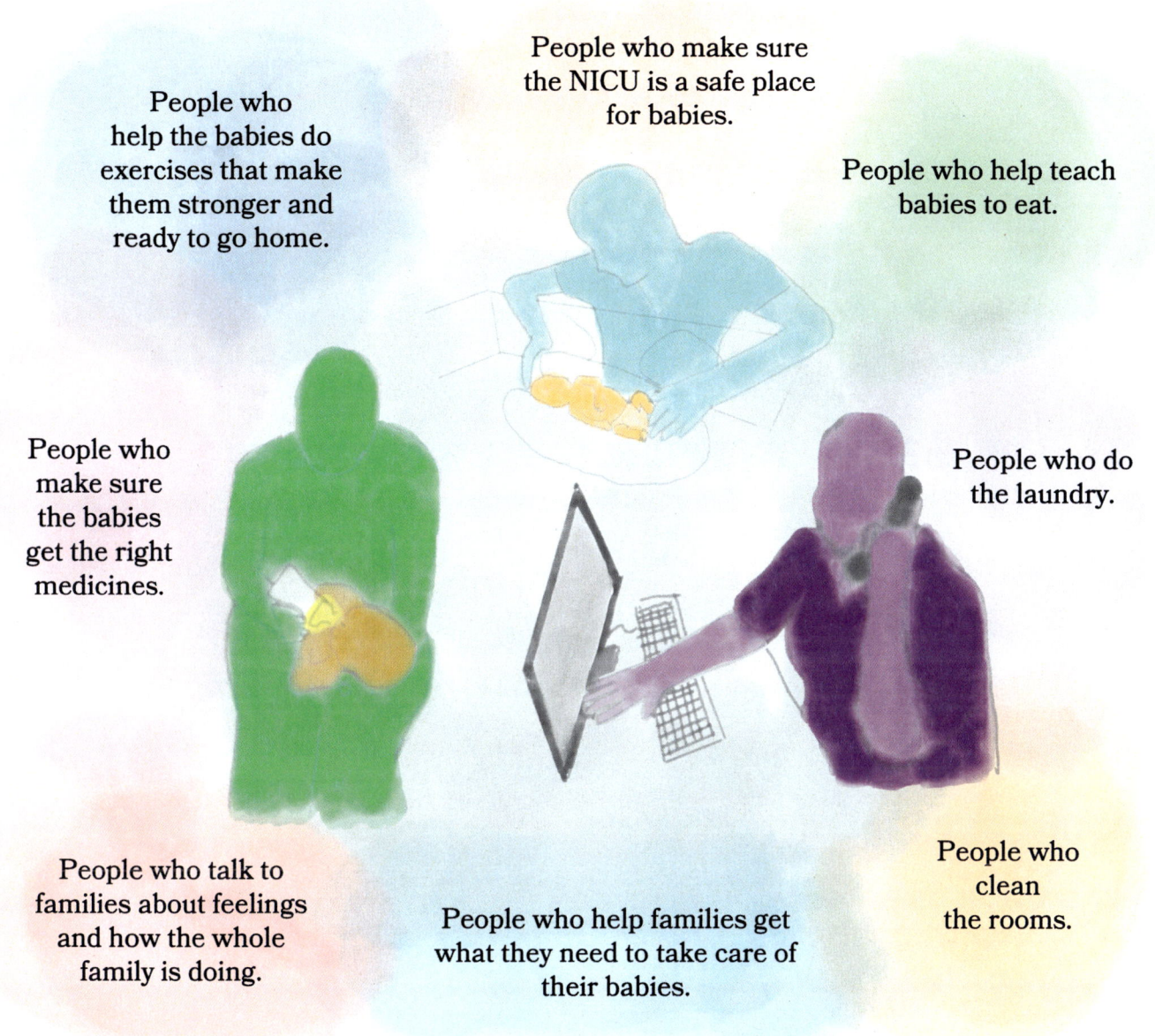

People who help the babies do exercises that make them stronger and ready to go home.

People who make sure the NICU is a safe place for babies.

People who help teach babies to eat.

People who make sure the babies get the right medicines.

People who do the laundry.

People who talk to families about feelings and how the whole family is doing.

People who help families get what they need to take care of their babies.

People who clean the rooms.

There are many people in the NICU that help take care of our new baby and help our family. Taking care of new babies takes lots of teamwork!

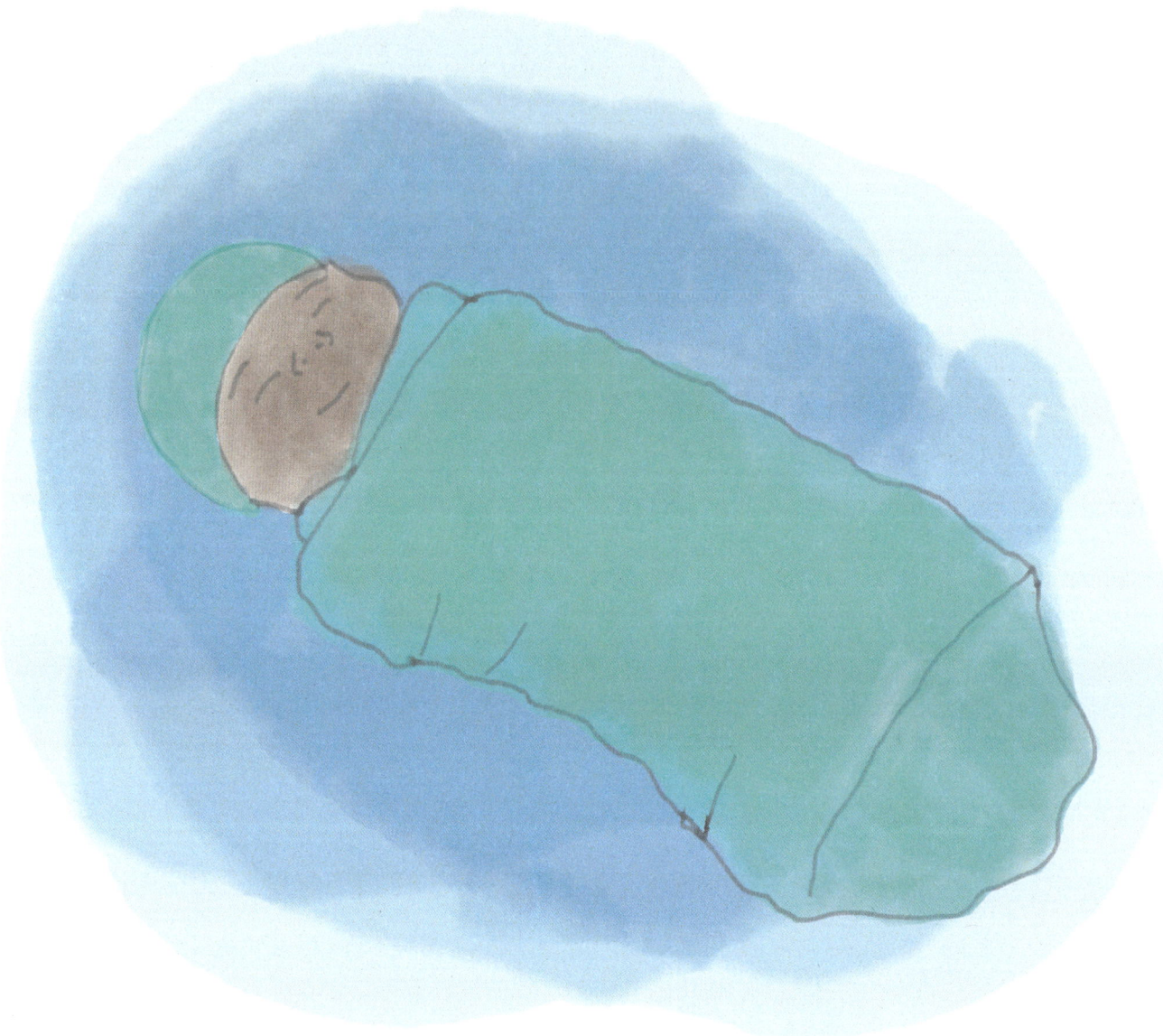

The NICU is a very quiet place. It's important for babies to get good rest. Good sleep helps babies' bodies grow and get healthier. When people are in the NICU, they have to use very quiet voices.

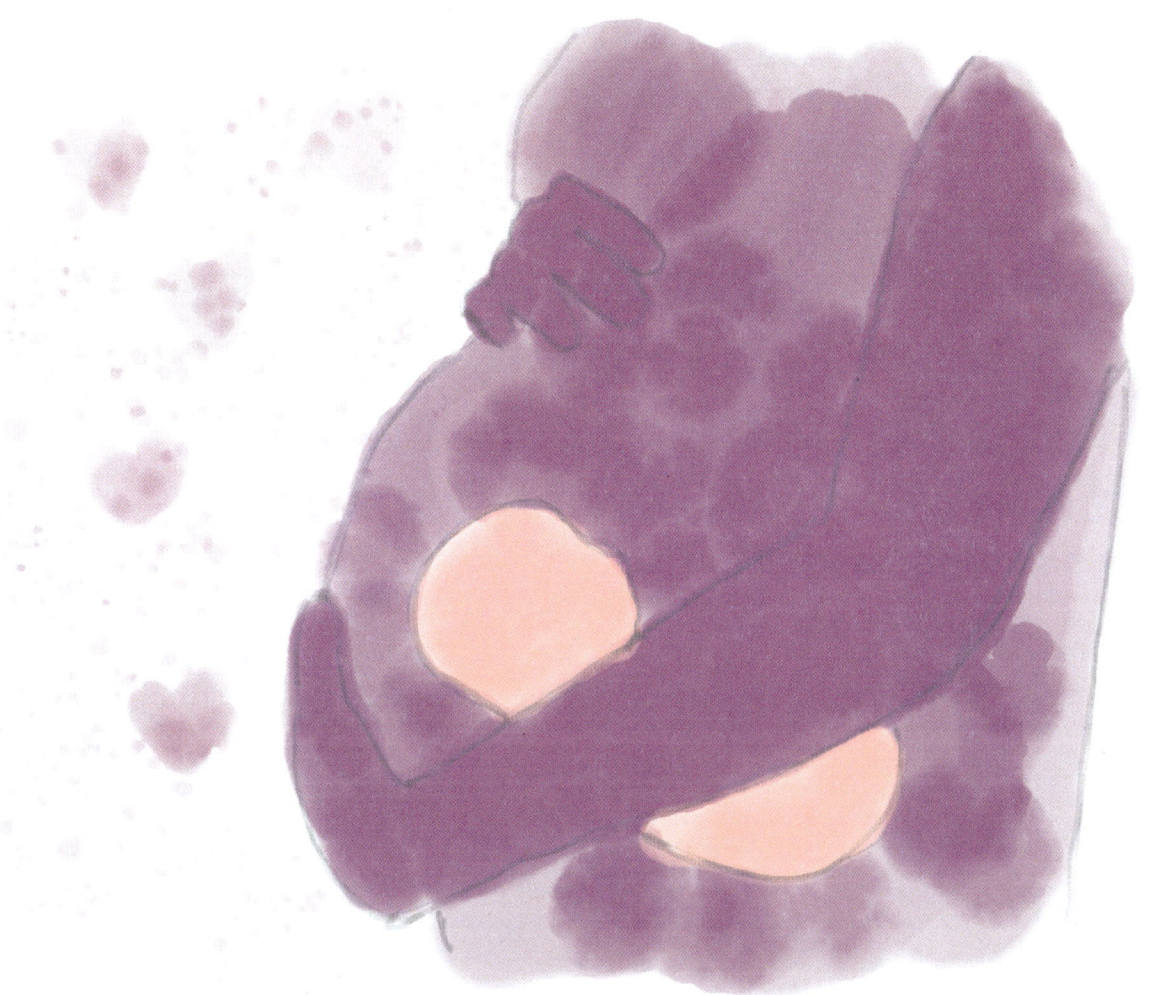

Some babies are in the NICU because they were born early. Most babies grow in their mommas' tummies for 9 months before they come out. 9 months is a long time, almost a year! There are babies in the NICU that came out 1, 2, 3, or even 4 months early. Lots of people call babies that are born early 'preemies' because they were born premature (a fancy word for early).

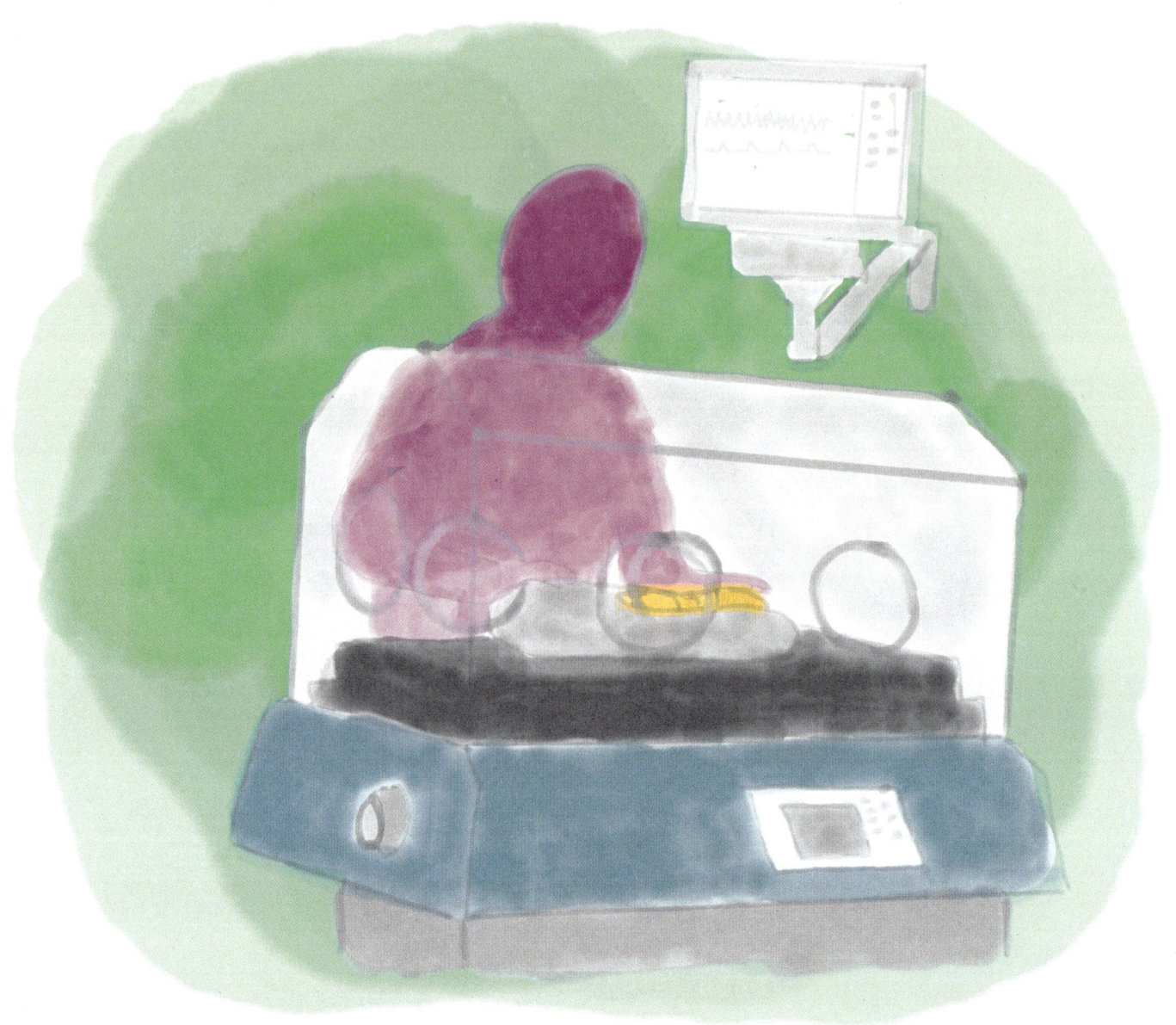

Preemies grow bigger during their time in the NICU. First, they have to sleep in a special cozy bed that feels dark, quiet, and warm, like they felt when they were inside their mommas' tummies. As they get bigger and can handle more light and noise, they get to switch to a crib.

Some babies are in the NICU for other reasons.

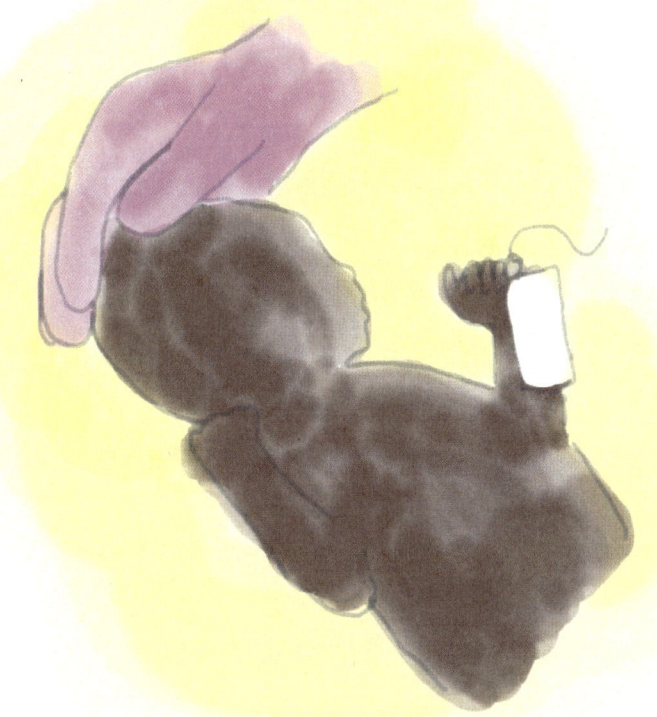

Some babies have an infection.

An infection means that they are sick and need medicine to fight the germs.

Some babies have jaundice.

Everyone has something called a liver that filters blood and removes the parts of the blood that the body is done using. Jaundice means that the baby's liver is having trouble doing this. It seems crazy, but there are special blue lights that help until the baby's liver can do the job on its own.

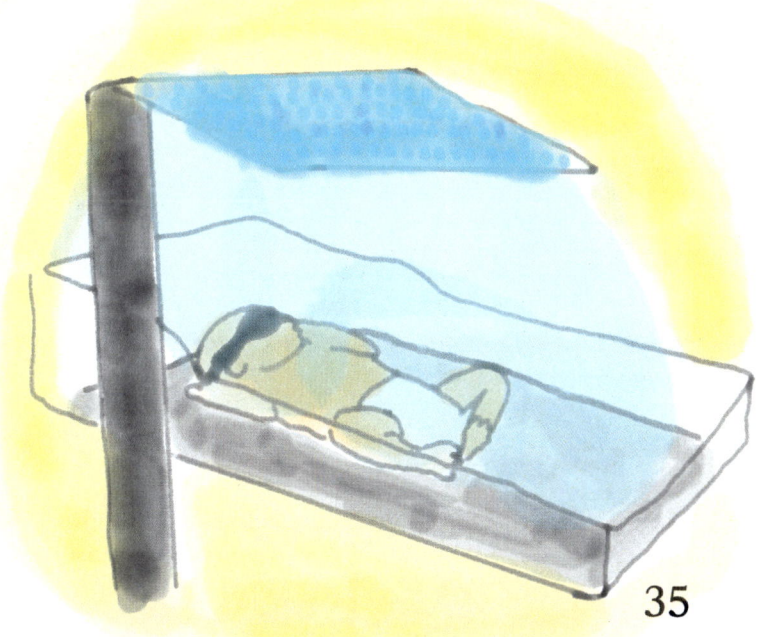

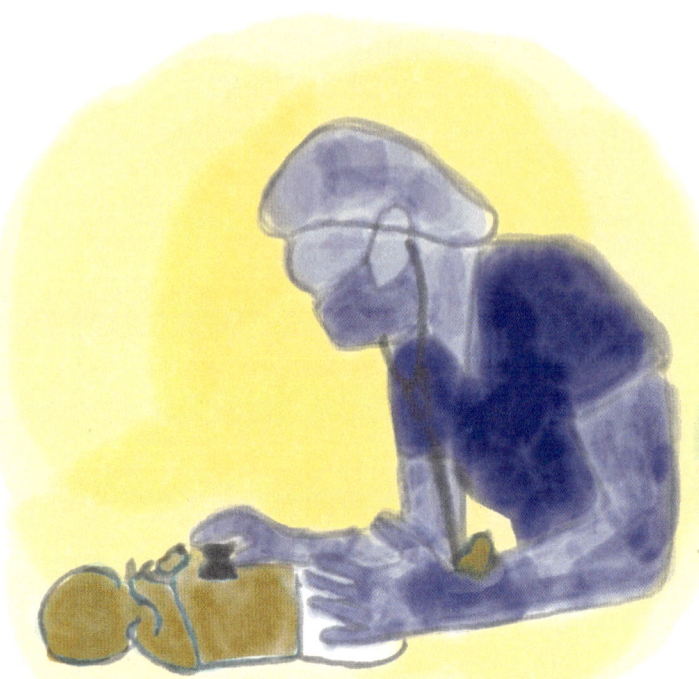

Some babies are in the NICU because when they grew inside their mommas, part of their body grew in a way that is different than most babies.

The baby can be checked by the doctors in the NICU, who are experts in babies. These doctors can help the baby's parent learn about whether the baby will need medicine, surgery, or special execises to help his or her body.

Some babies in the NICU just need to be watched extra carefully to make sure they are healthy.

Since babies can't talk, they can't tell us when something is wrong. Certain things a baby does may make us wonder if they need extra help. Having doctors and nurses watch the baby and check his or her blood, breathing, and eating can tell us if the baby needs extra help.

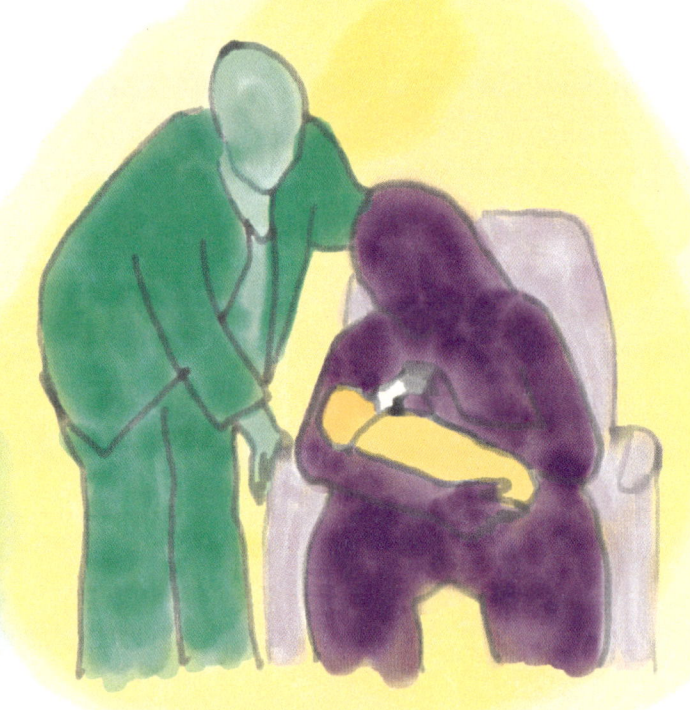

36

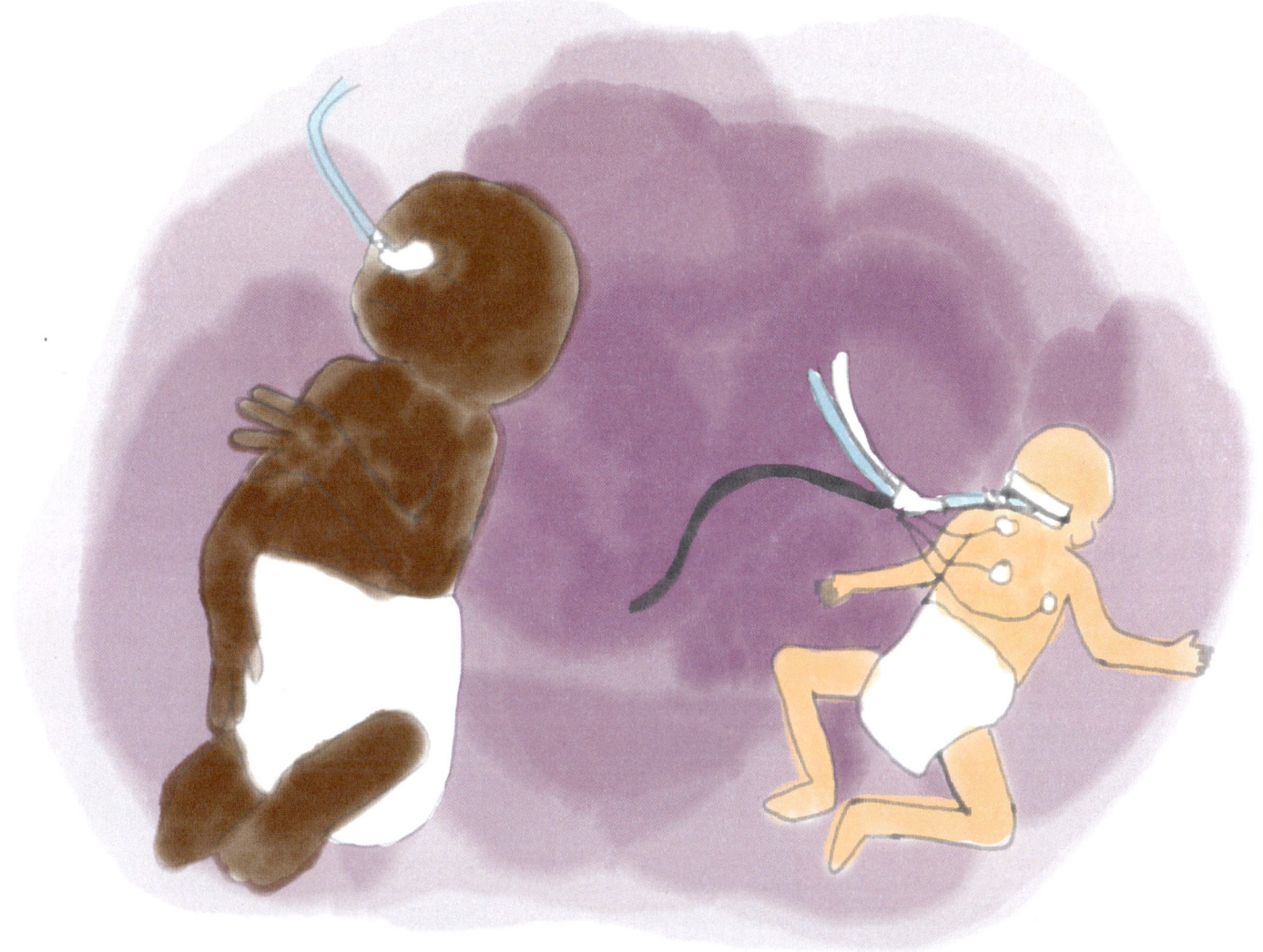

Some babies need help breathing until they are ready to breathe on their own. A baby can get extra oxygen to breathe through a tube that rests in front of his or her nose. If a baby needs more help breathing, a tube can be put in the baby's mouth. This tube is connected to a machine called a ventilator that helps the baby breathe.

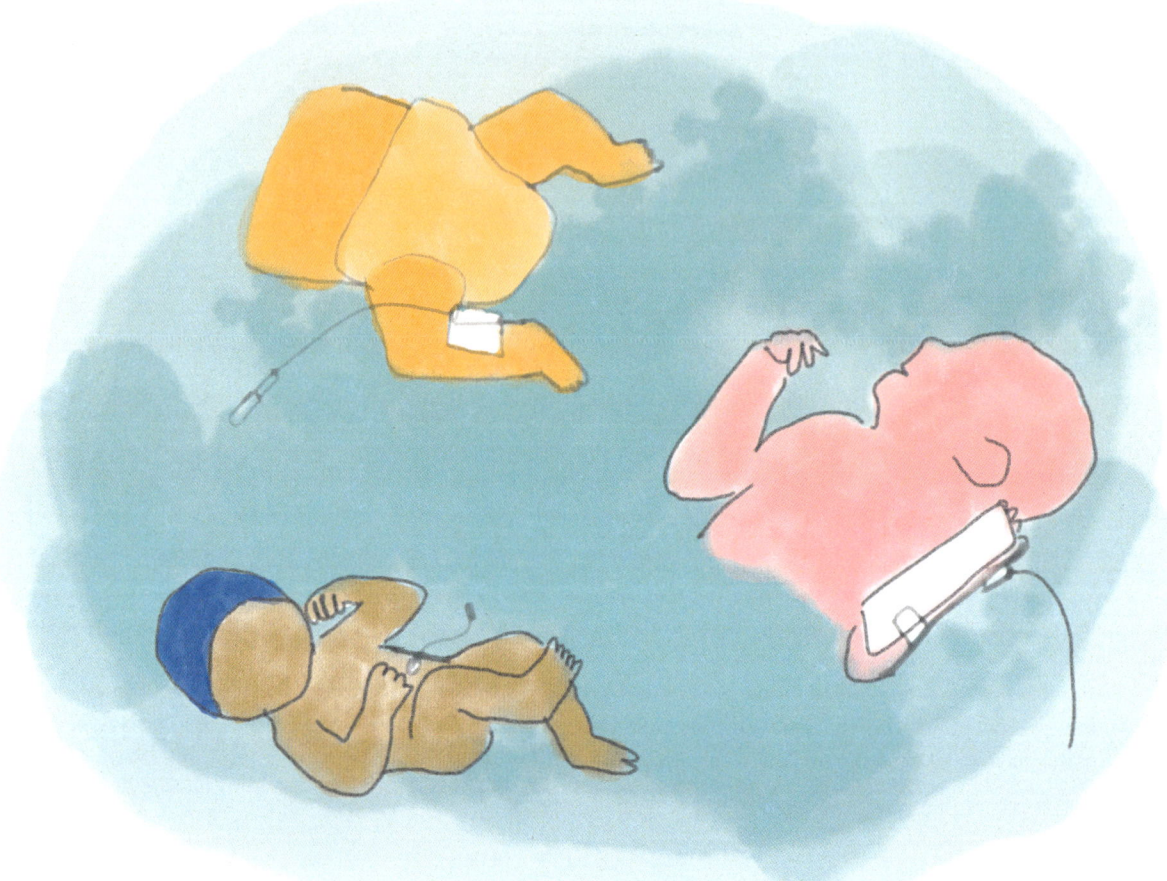

Many babies also get an IV. An IV is a small tube that goes into the baby's body and is used to give the baby medicine. This tube might go into their belly button when they are first born (also callede a UVC). Most of the time, the IV tube is on the baby's hand, foot, arm, or head. IVs might hurt for a few seconds, when they are first put in, but once they are there, they do not hurt the baby. Sometimes, babies that need an IV for more than a few days get something called a PICC line instead. PICC lines can last for weeks or even months and are much harder for the baby to accidently pull out.

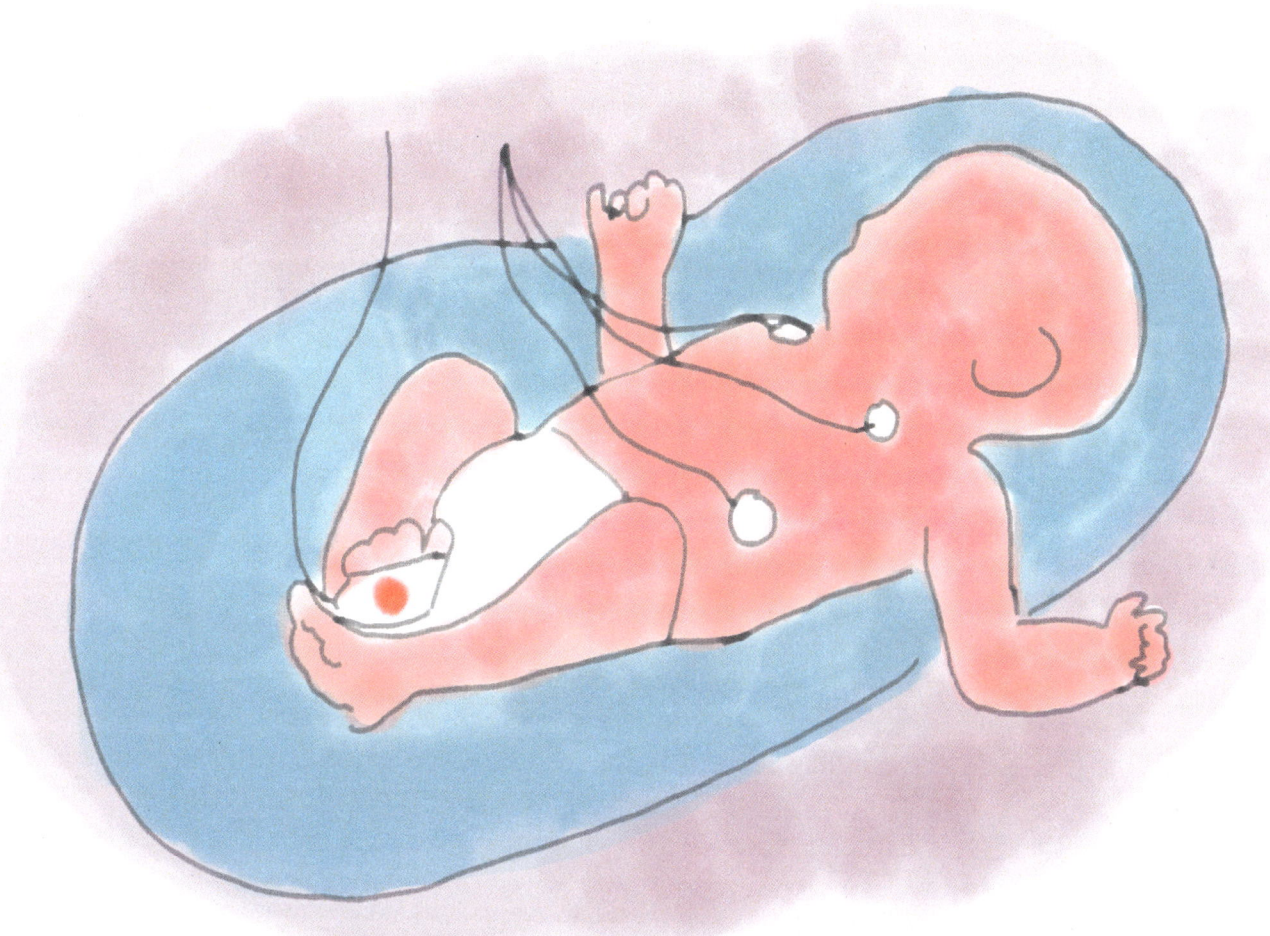

While babies are in the NICU, the nurses and doctors watch them closely. They pay attention to how well each baby is breathing and how quickly the baby's heart is beating. The baby wears three special stickers on his or her chest and stomach. There is also a small red light that is attached to the baby's foot. These stickers and light are connected to a computer, and the computers show the nurses and doctors how the baby is doing.

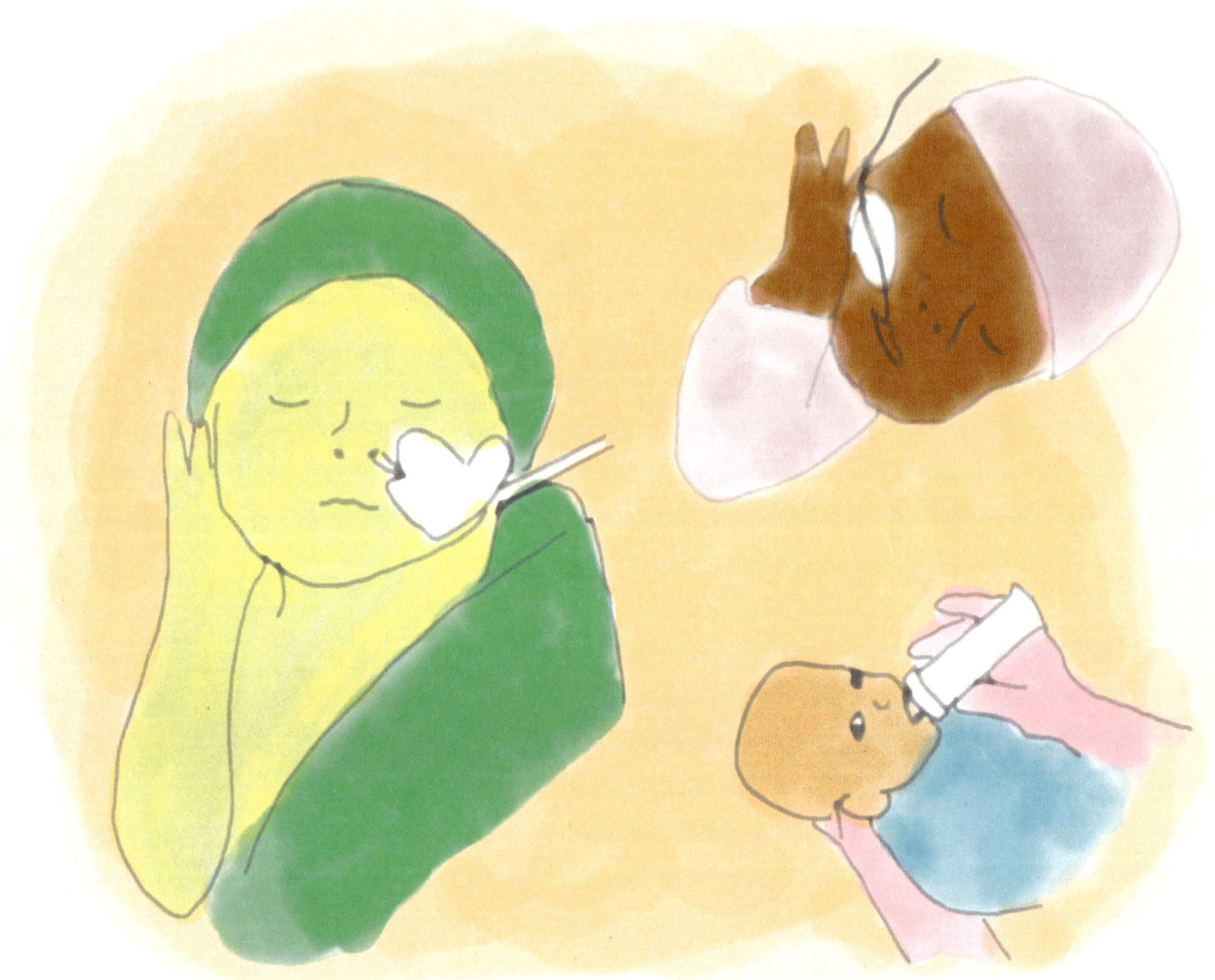

Many babies in the NICU are not ready to drink milk because their bodies are too sick or they were born too early. The nurses can give the baby milk through another small tube in the baby's nose or mouth. As the baby gets bigger and healthier, the baby usually gets better at figuring out how to drink. The baby's nurses and parents can help them learn, but sometimes, it can take a long time!

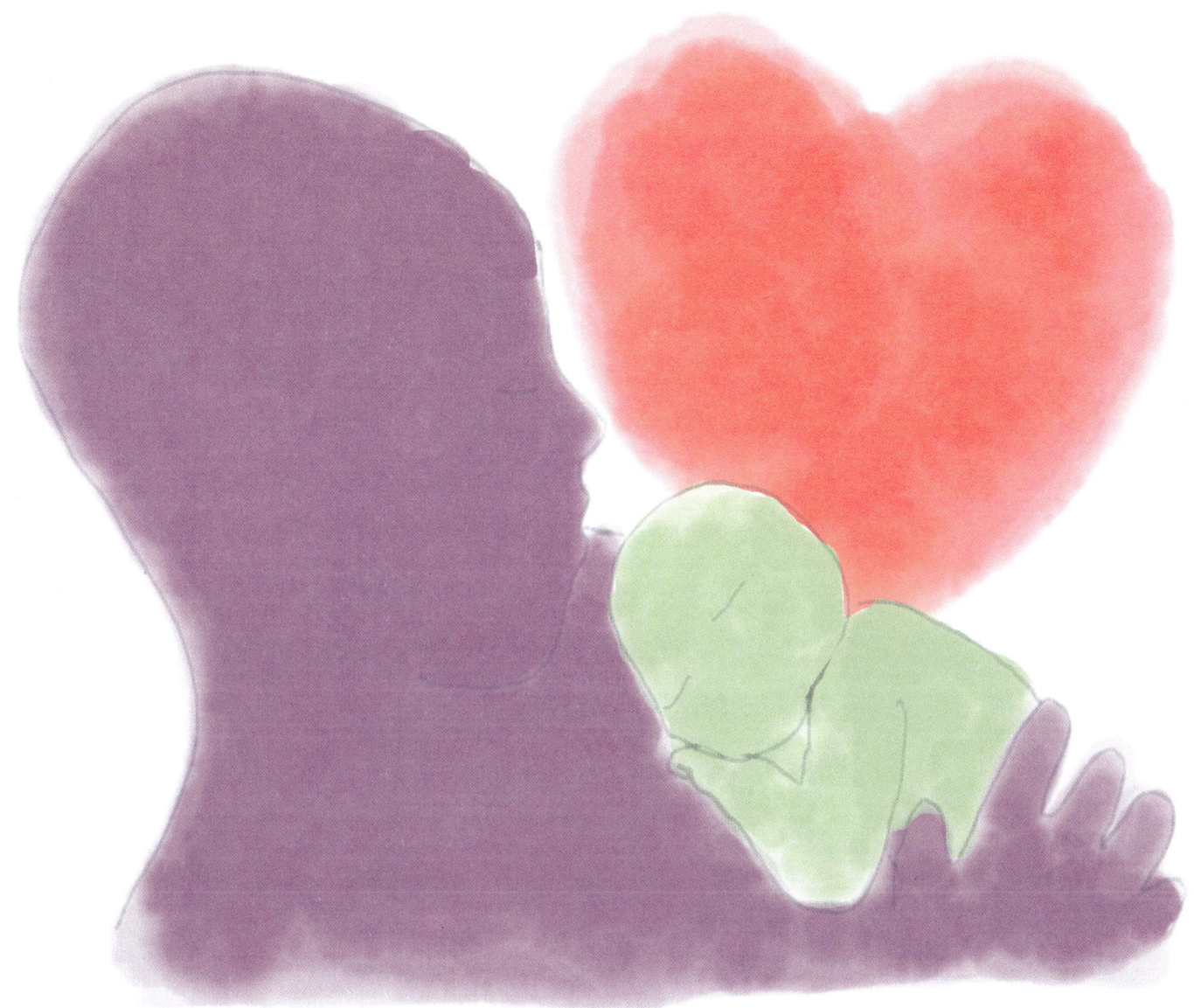

While our new baby is in the hospital, it is important for the adults in our family to go to the hospital and help take care of our baby. They can hold the baby to help the baby feel good. They can help the baby practice drinking milk.

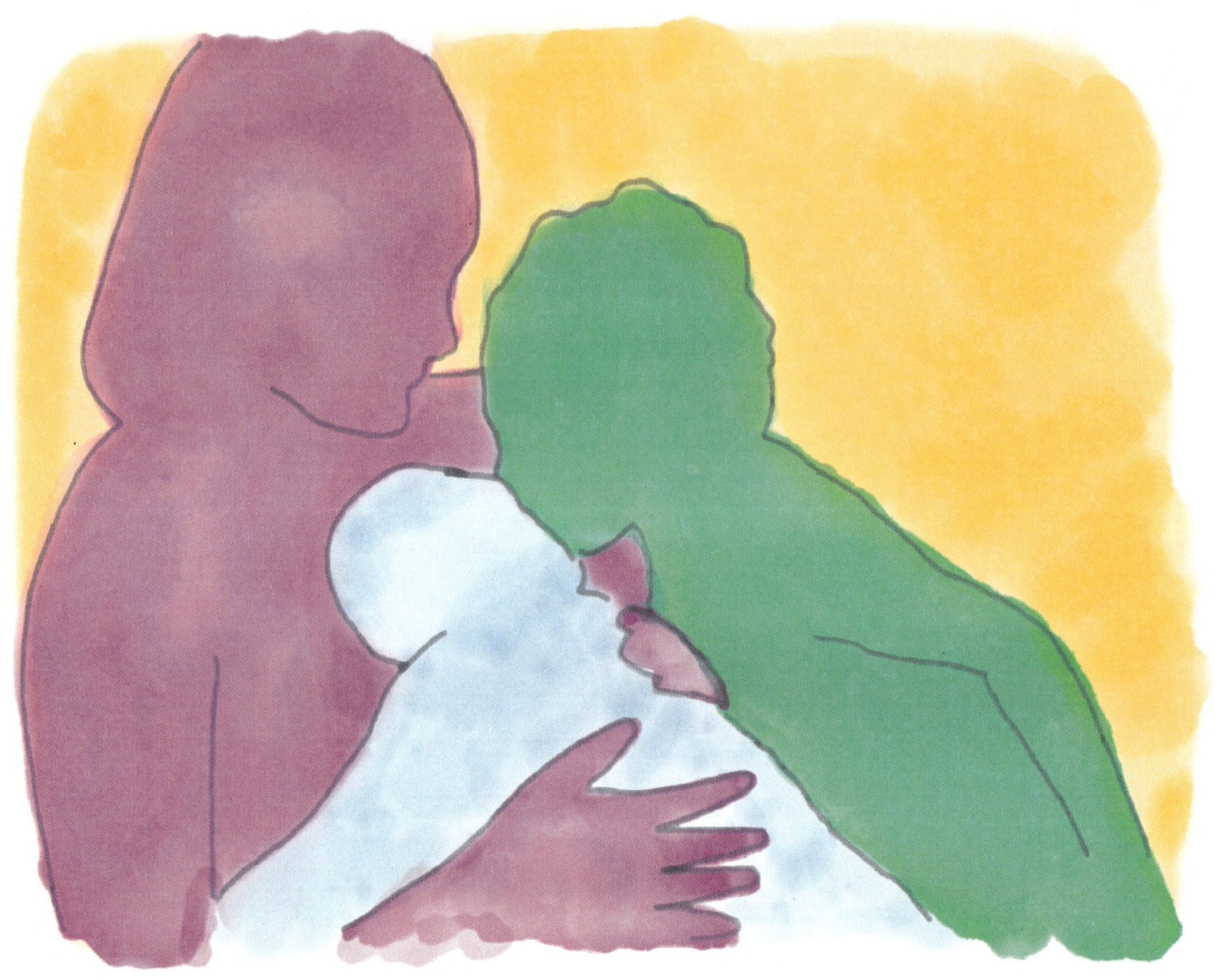

I wish that our whole family could be together. When our baby is healthy and can drink enough milk, our baby will come home. I can help take care of our baby. There are all sorts of things the new baby will need help with. I will find things that I am good at helping with.

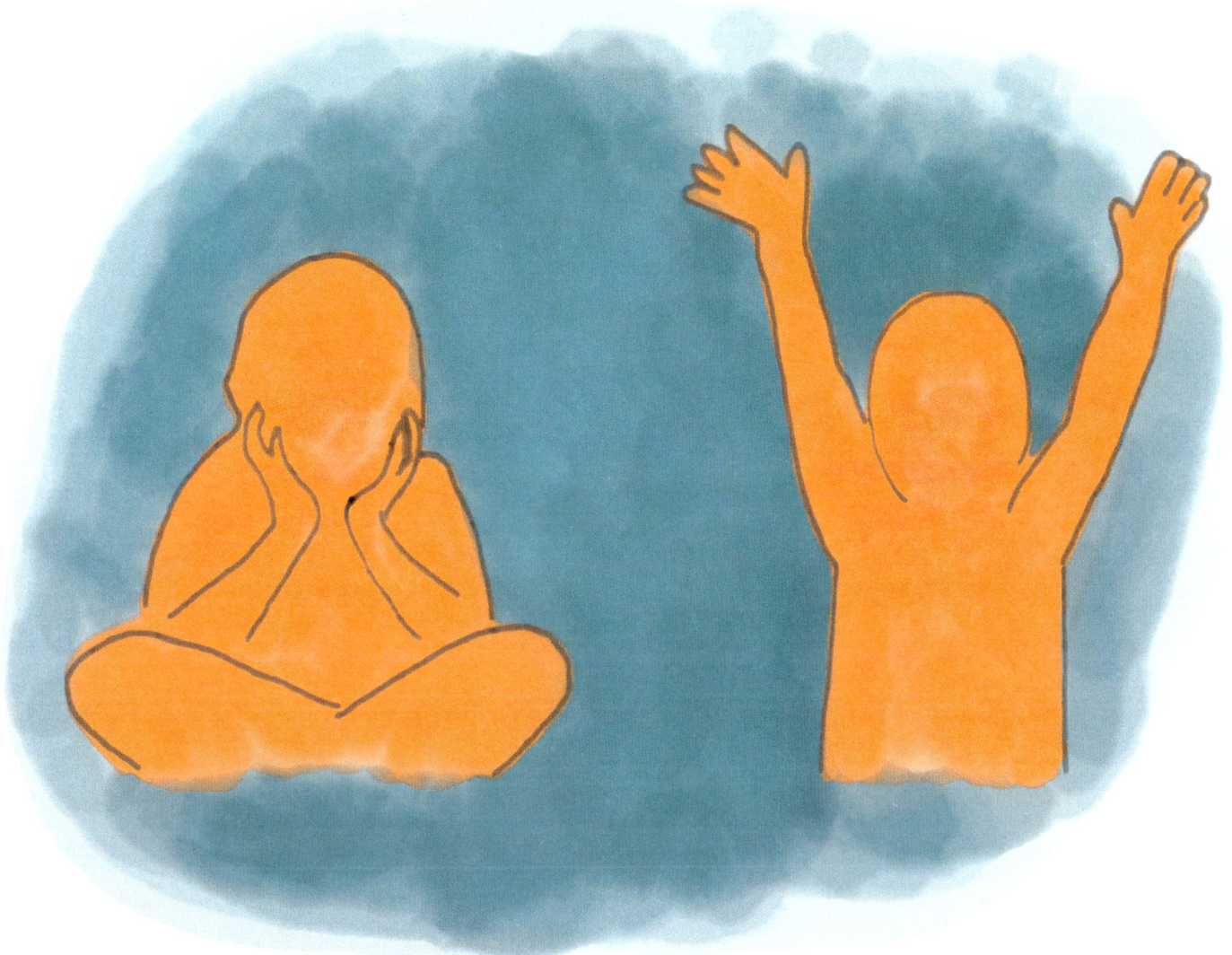

Being a new brother or sister , I might have lots of new feelings. I might feel excited that the new baby is finally here. I might feel sad that the baby has to stay at the hospital. Sometimes, I might feel jealous that people are focused on the baby. All of those feelings are okay. I can talk to my family about them.

43

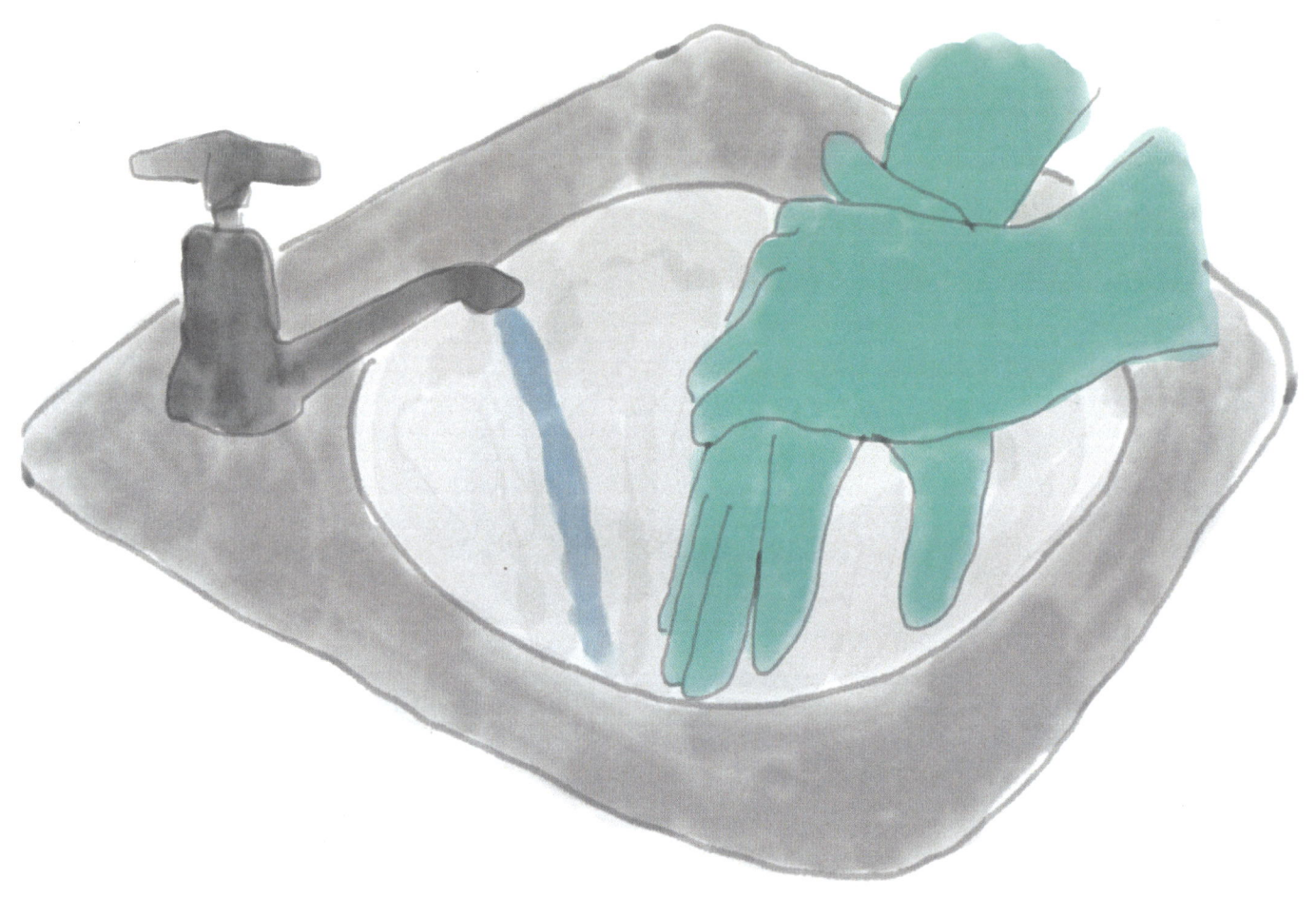

We will be extra careful about germs to help keep our baby healthy.
We will wash our hands before we hold our baby. At the hospital, the
doctors and nurses wash their hands before they touch our baby.

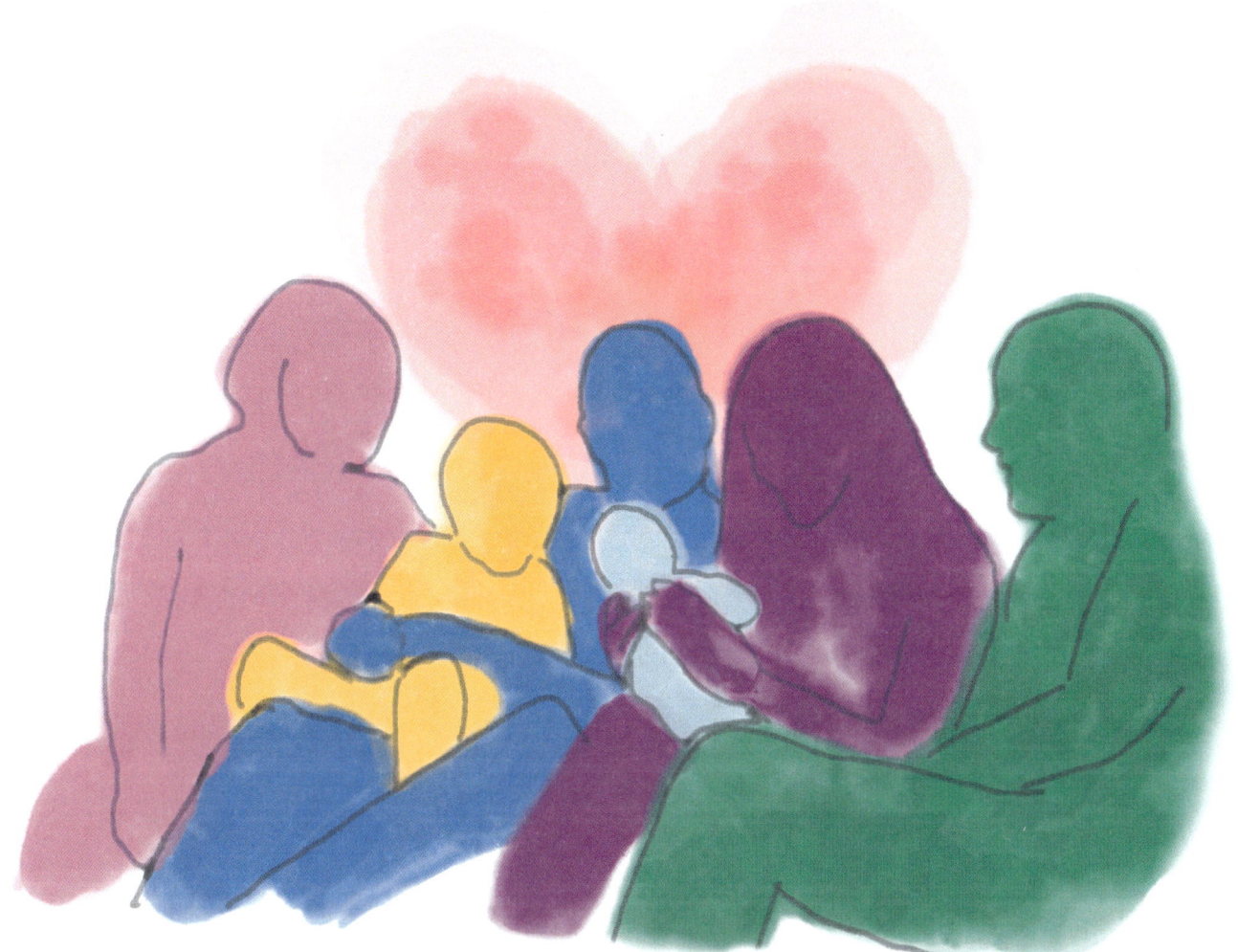

Brother and sisters can be helpful even while their baby is in the NICU. They can show their love by making artwork for the baby and sending it to the hospital or putting it by the baby's crib for when they come home. Brothers and sisters can also help by trying to be patient when their parent has to be at the hospital to help the baby. Parents love all of their kids and might feel sad that they can't be with all of them at the same time. Brothers and sisters can give their parent big hugs to help them feel good during this hard time.

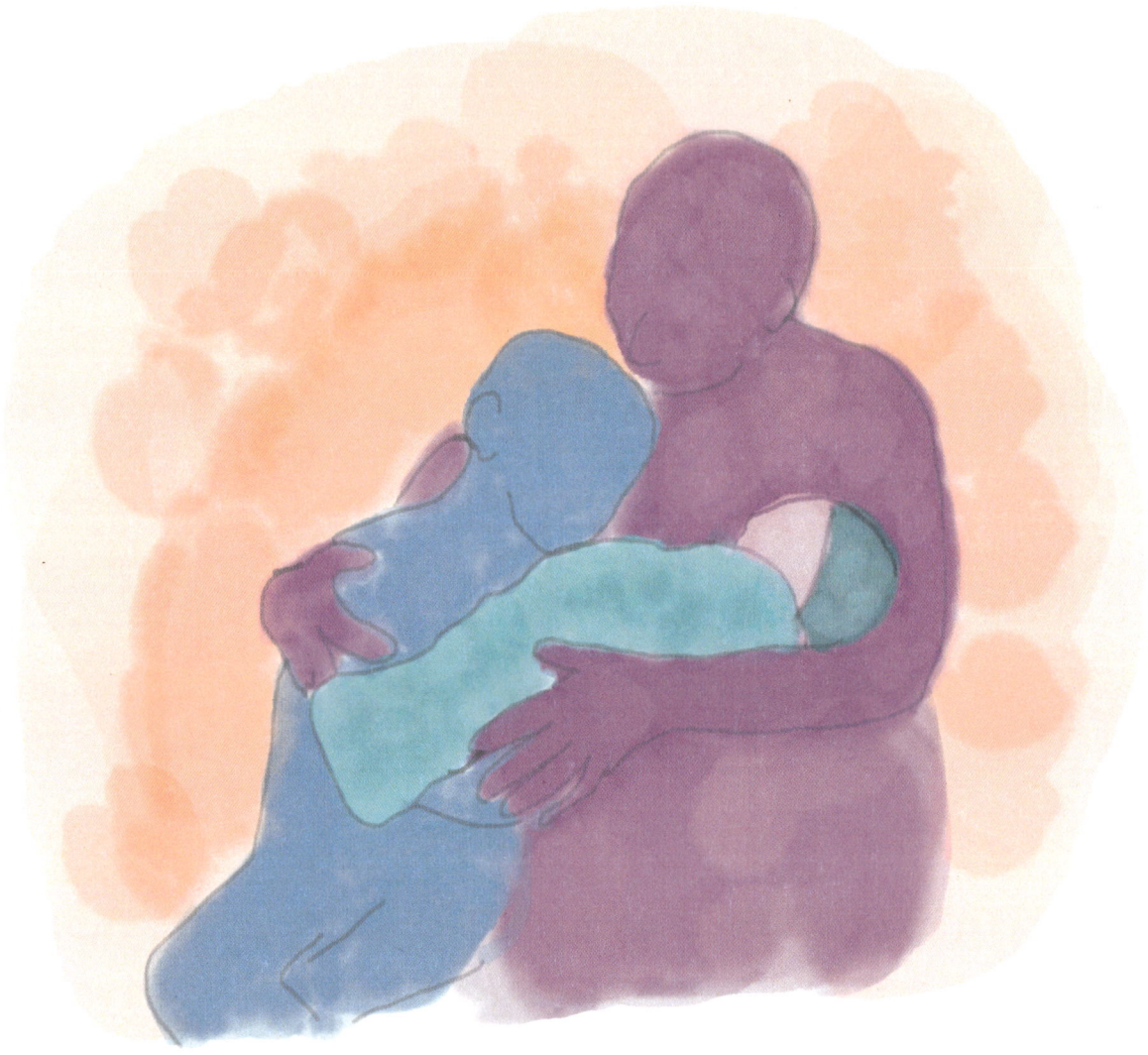

When the baby comes home, there are many other jobs brothers and sisters can do. They can help get diapers for the baby and help pick out what clothes the baby will wear. They can tell the baby stories or read a book to the baby. They can try to be patient because their parent will need to help them and the new baby.

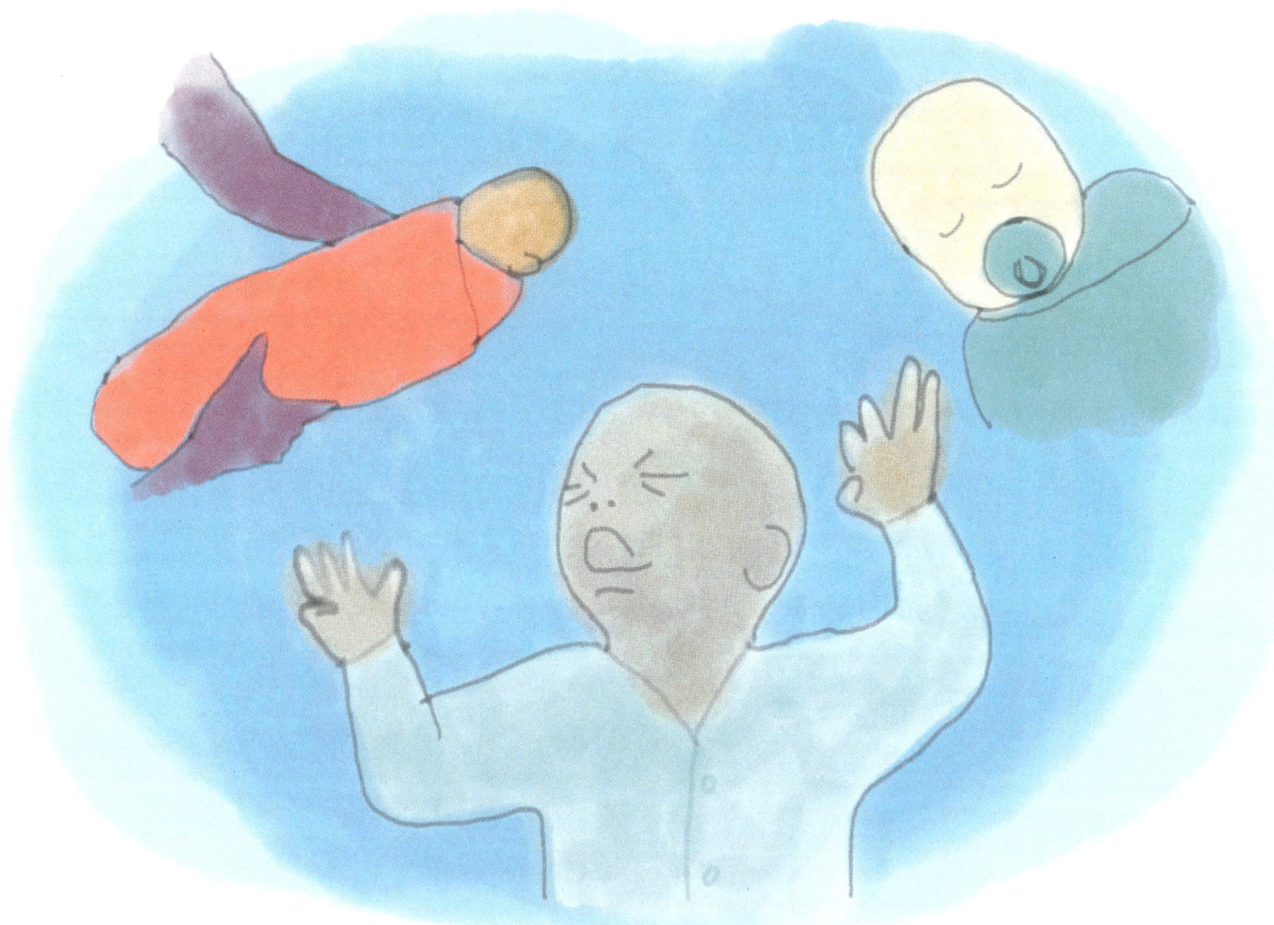

Sometimes, babies cry. When our baby comes home, our baby will cry to tell us that he or she is hungry, tired, or uncomfortable. Sometimes, it is hard to figure out how to make a baby feel more comfortable. Some babies like to suck on a pacifier or their fingers to feel calm. Many new babies feel comfortable when they are wrapped up in a blanket. My parent will try to help our baby feel good, but sometimes, the baby might still cry. If the baby's crying is too loud or it bothers me, I can go into a different room and take a break from the crying. Crying is okay. Taking a break is okay too.

47

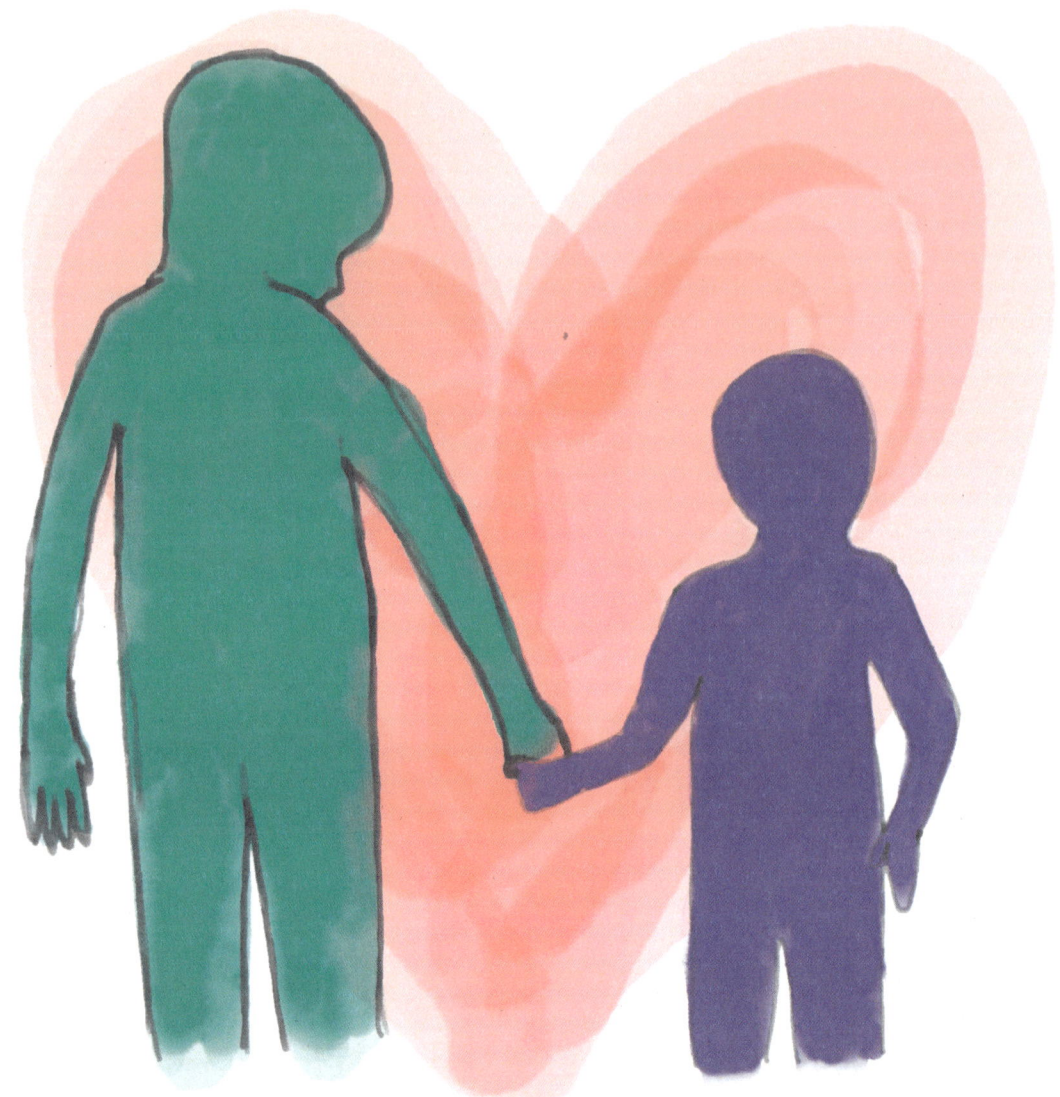

Being a NICU brother or sister is special. It means I am a part of a family who takes extra special care of our baby. As our baby grows, it may be hard to remember this time when our baby had to stay at the hospital. Someday, I can tell my sibling all about when they were brand new and lived in the NICU.

Keep talking! Here are some more questions that you and your whole family can discuss.

(Of course, you can come up with your own questions too!)

What tubes does our baby have?

Has anyone noticed things that our baby really likes or doesn't like?

If I feel sad or upset about our baby being the NICU, it might help to talk about it. If my parent isn't around, who is someone else I can talk to when I am feeling upset?

What is my 'birth story'? Did I have to stay in the NICU too?

What was I like as a baby?

Do other people in my family know their birth stories?
We are all special and different!

What questions do you have for your baby's doctors and nurses?

(Write them down below so that you don't forget. Have your parents ask for you or if you get to visit, ask them yourself!)

I Love You Everywhere and All of the Time

A NICU Read Aloud Book

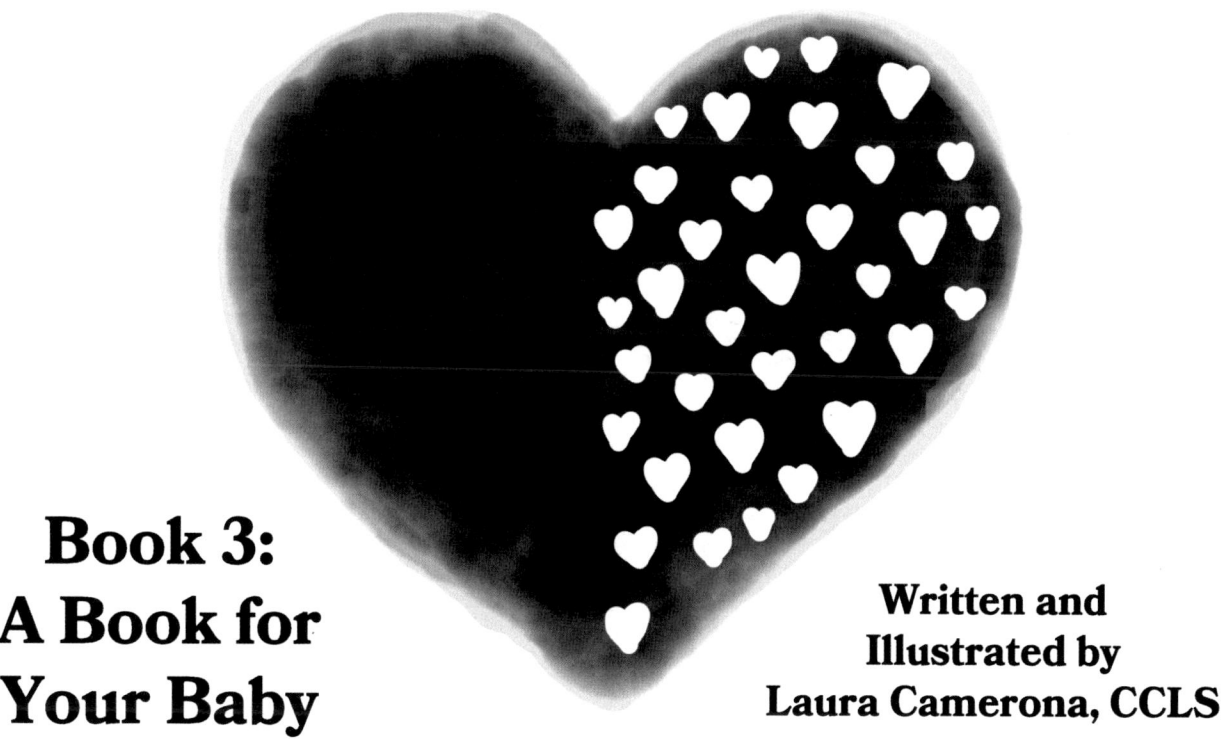

**Book 3:
A Book for
Your Baby**

**Written and
Illustrated by
Laura Camerona, CCLS**

Reading to babies is good for their brains. Your baby was listening to voices when he or she was in utero. It is part of how the human brain develops. As your baby continues to develop, you can help that development by exposing your baby to the rhythmic and steady speech that comes from reading a book. In addition, reading to your baby helps he or she feel connected to you! If you are in a situation that keeps you from being able to hold your baby, reading can be special bonding for both of you.

This book was created to offer pages with high contrast pictures for your baby as his or her vision develops. The text is simple and easy for big siblings to read as well. If a sibling isn't able to visit the NICU, you can try recording the sibling reading this or another book and playing it for the baby at a low volume!

If your baby is sensitive to sounds and visual stimulation, read with a very quiet voice and watch for signs of overstimulation (such as yawning, spreading fingers, sneezing. and fussiness).

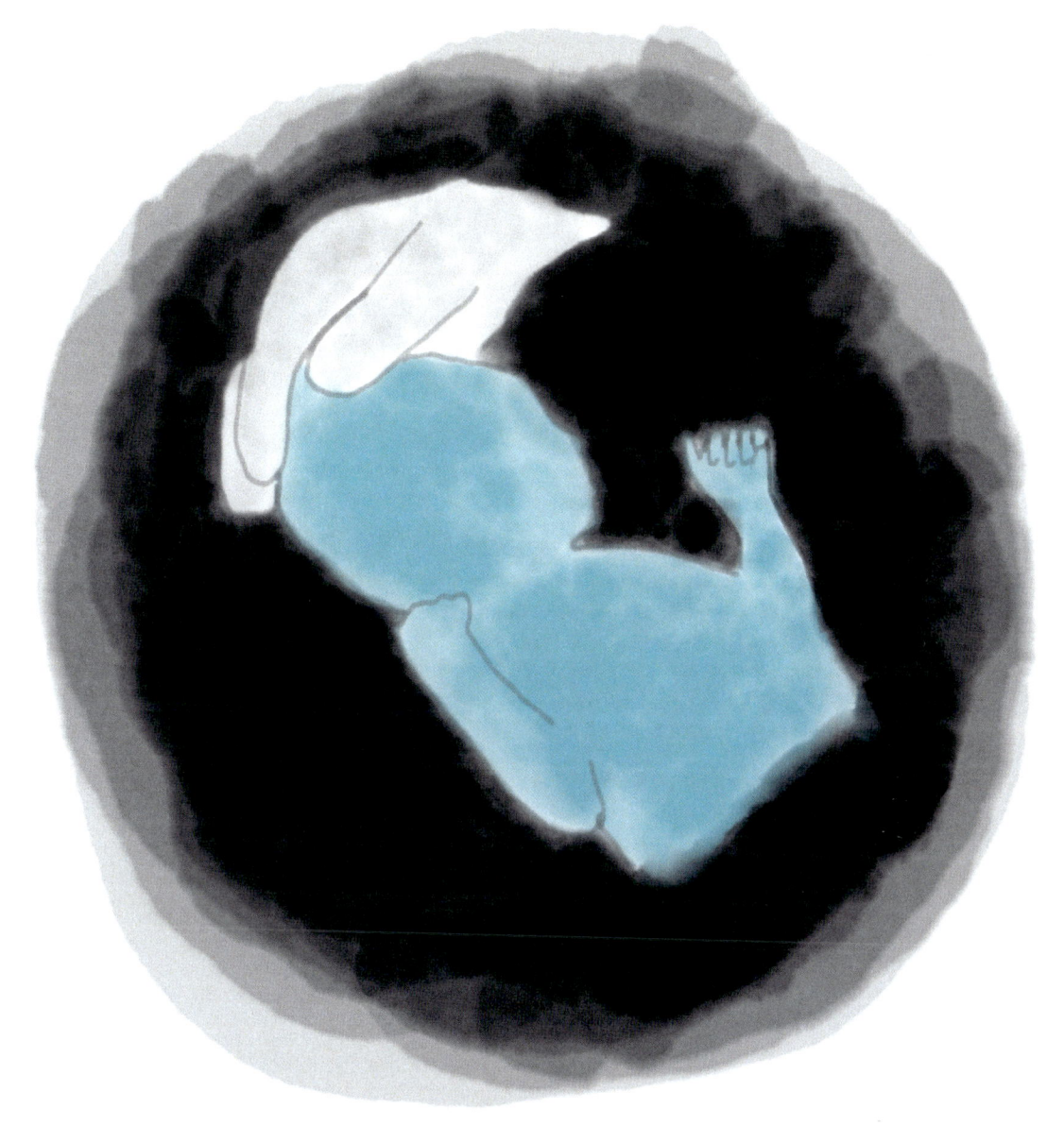

Sweet little baby of mine. You are perfect.
You are you.

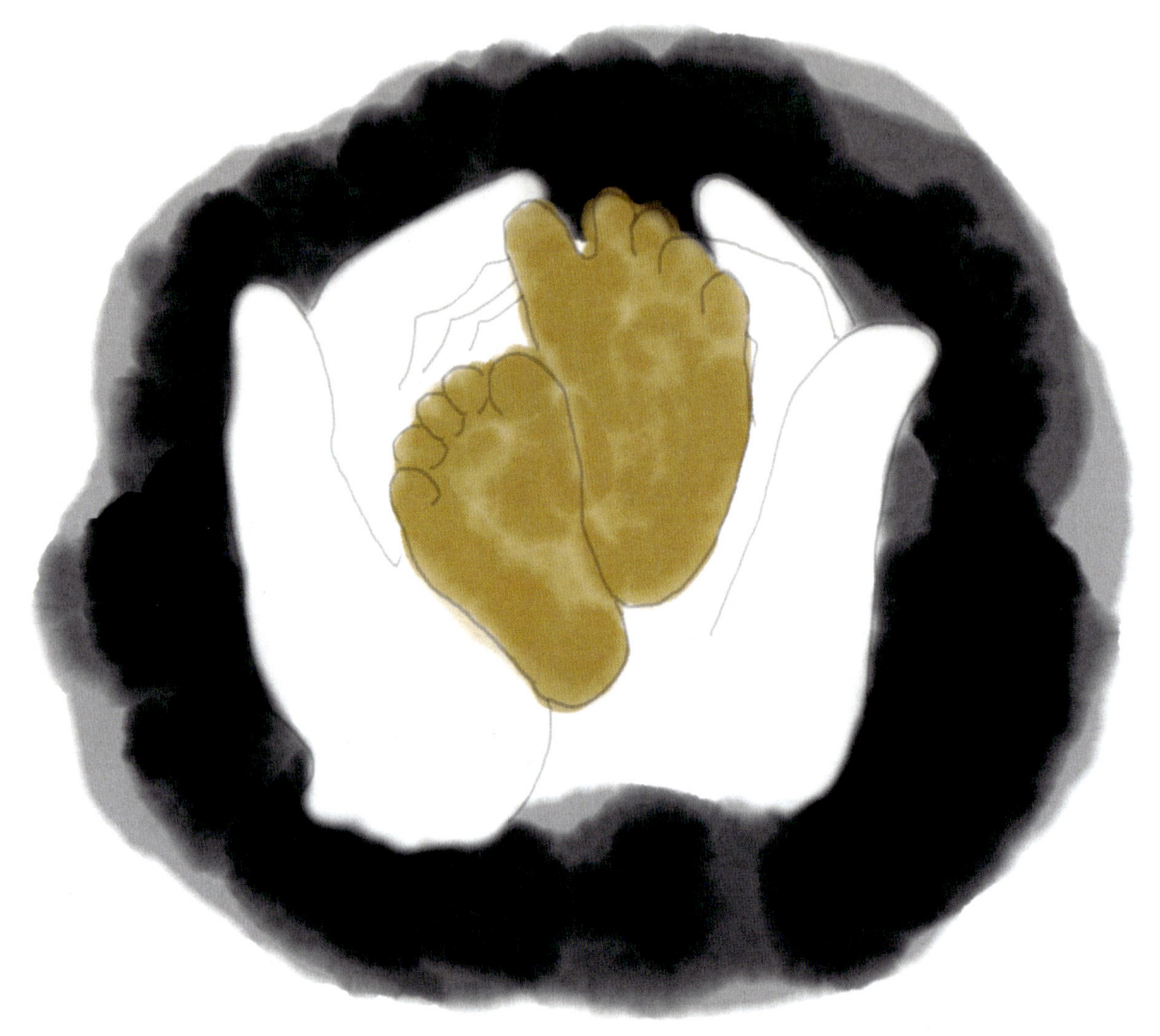

I love everything about you. Your fingers, your
toes, your eyes, your tiny nose....

(Add more things you love about your baby.)

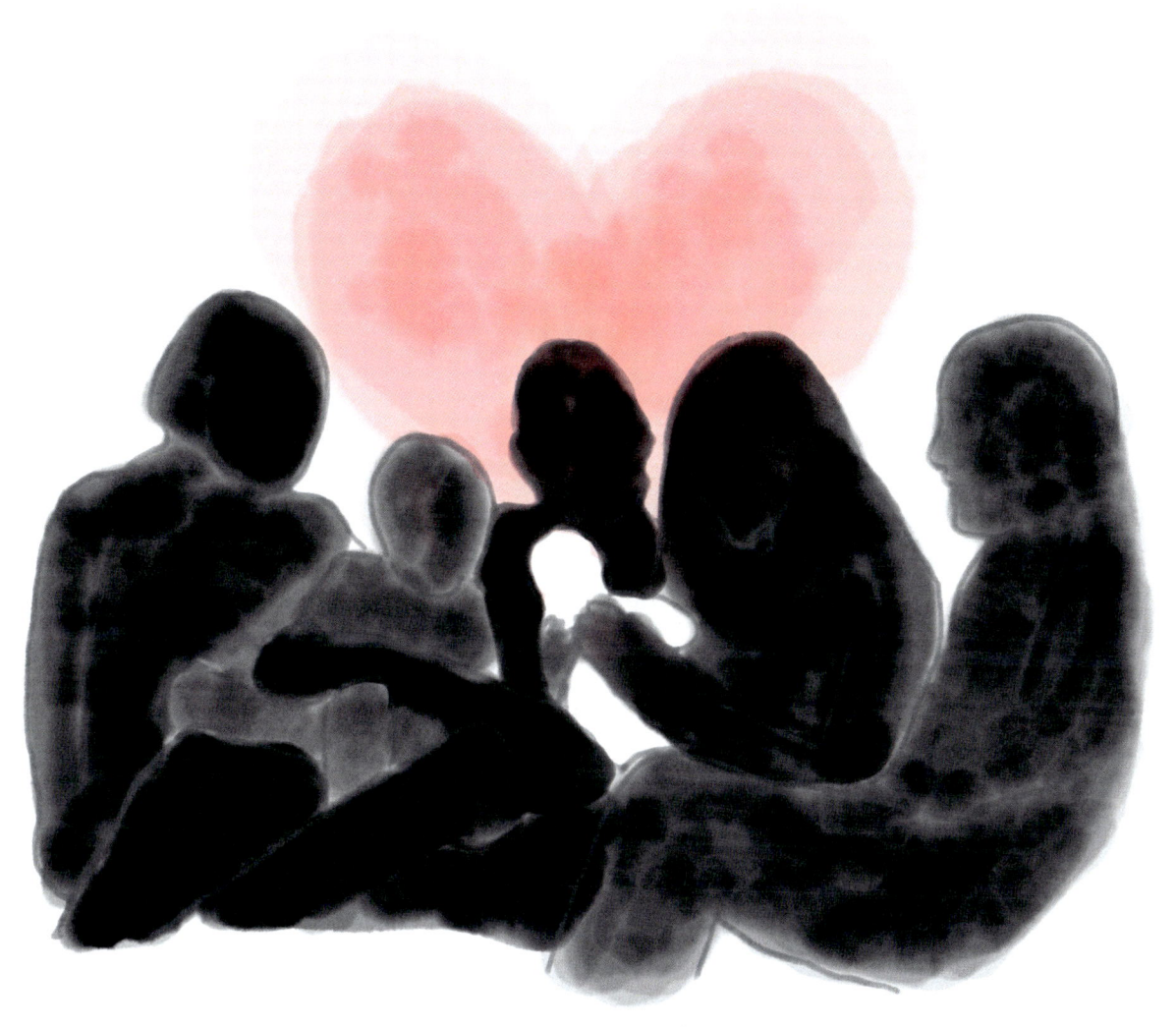

You belong with me. You are a part of us.
Soon, we will take you home.

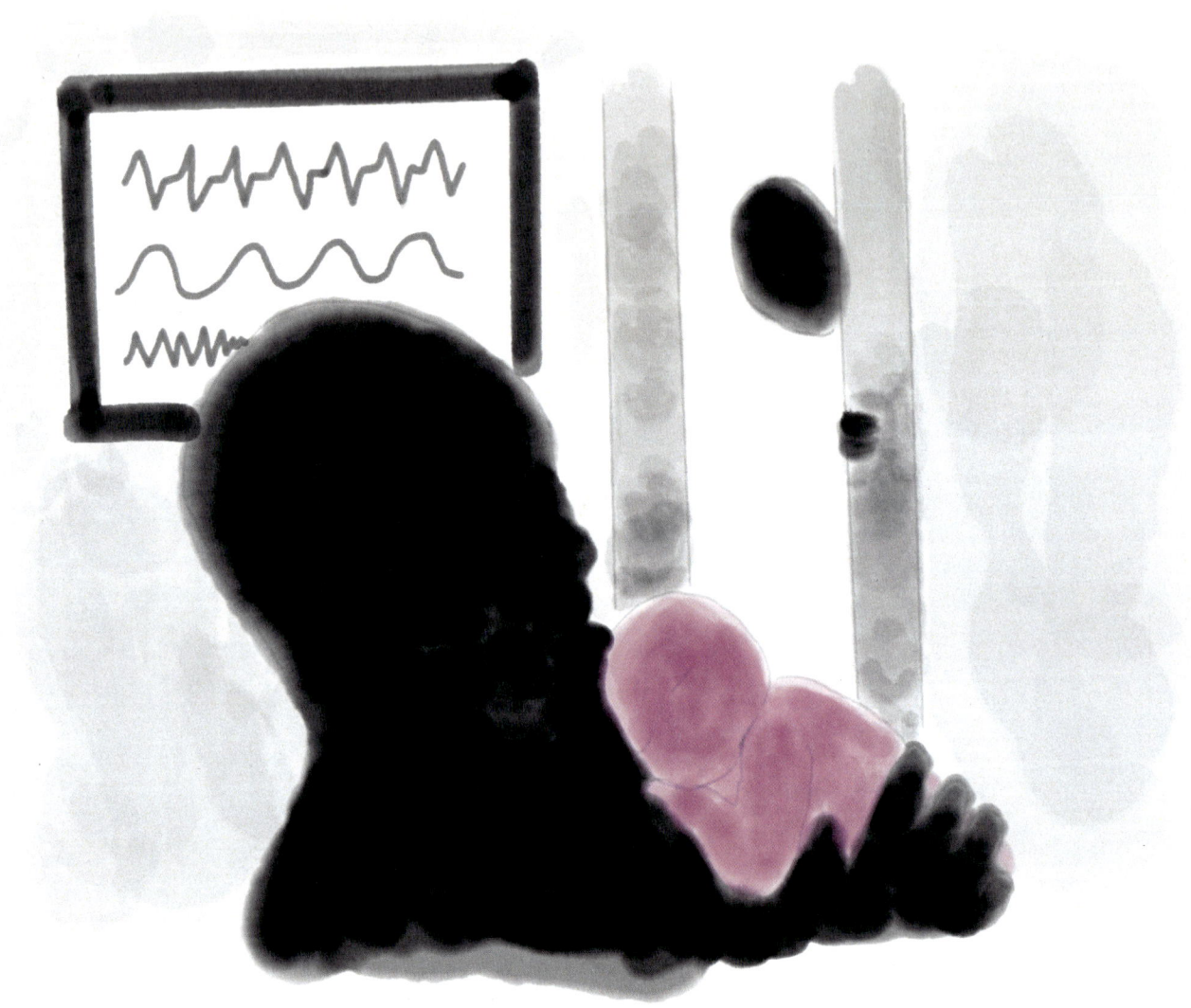

Home will be the very best. We will be together, away from the beeps and the opening and closing door.

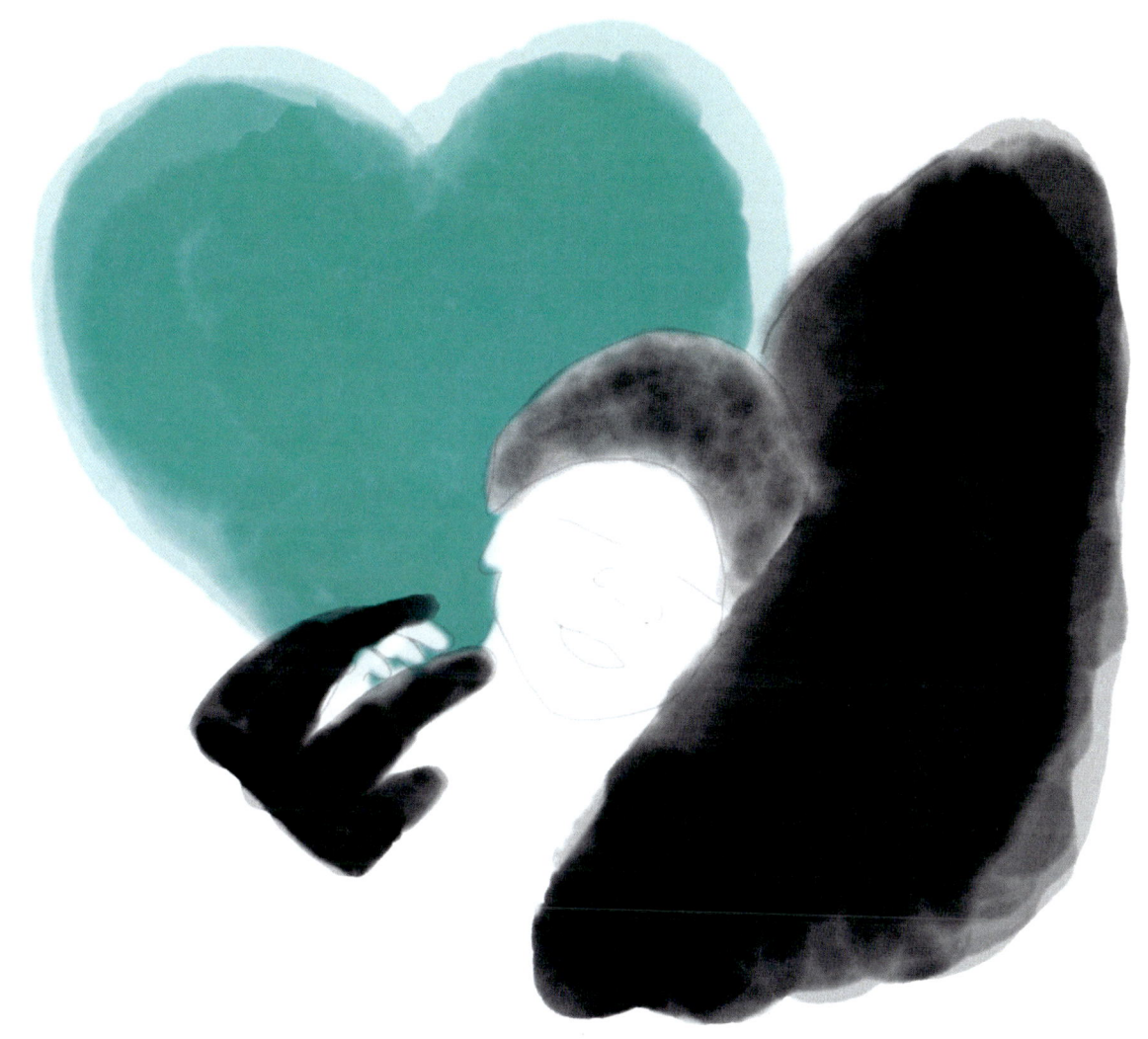

We will snuggle, and I will take sweet pictures
of you trying your first food or flashing
a new smile.

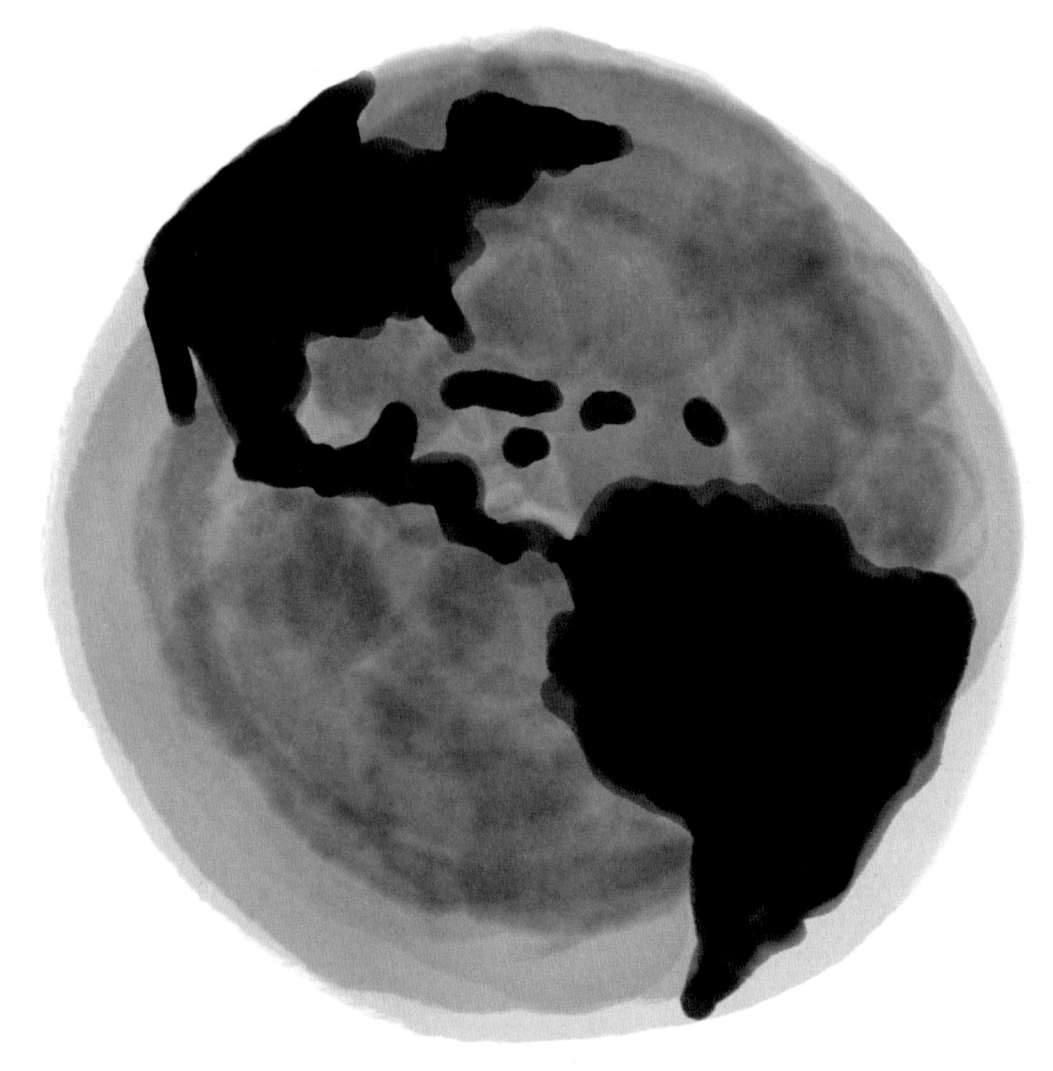

Someday, we will adventure. I will show you
new things and new places.

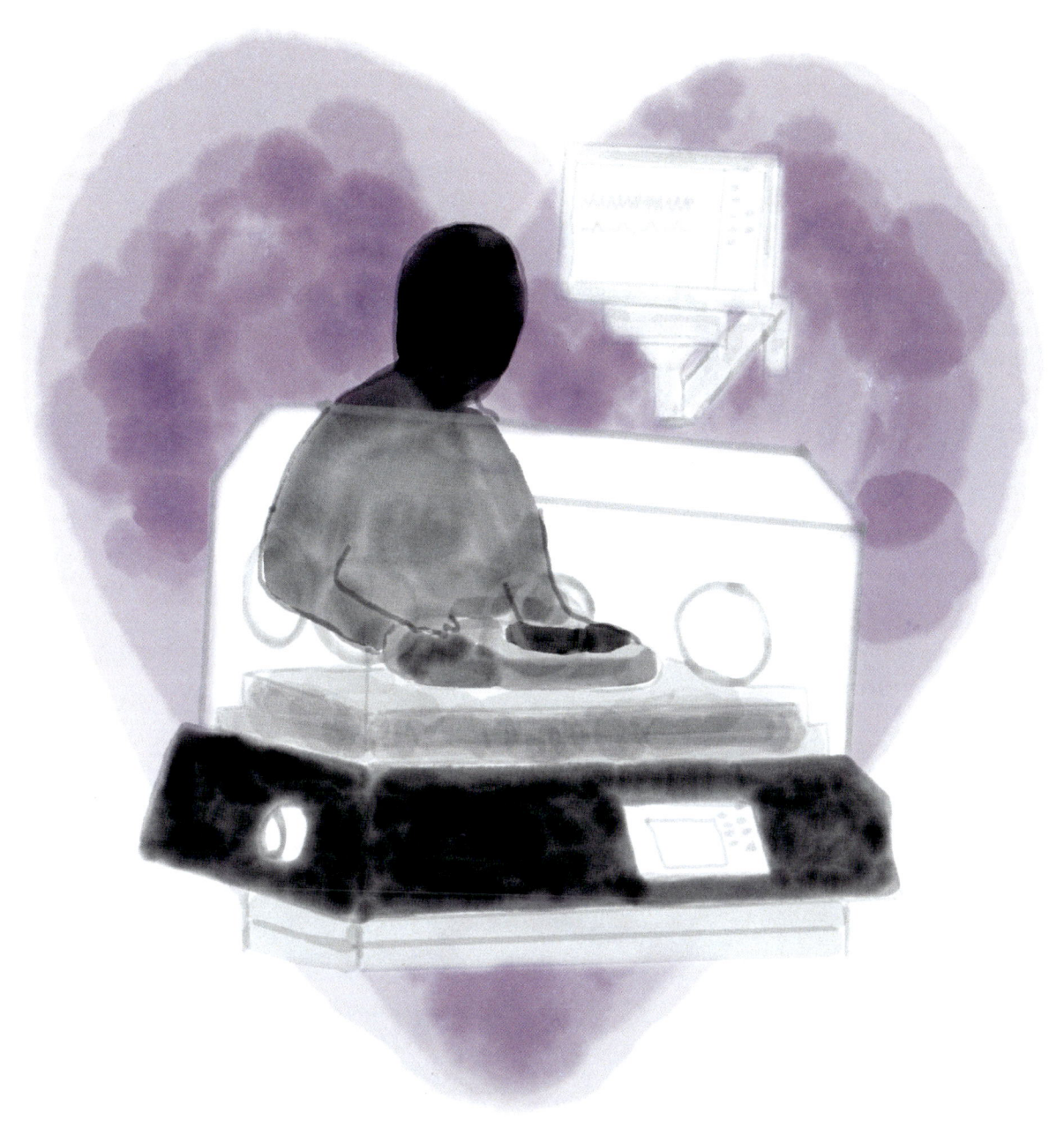

But for now, I will love you right here.

I love you everywhere and all of the time.

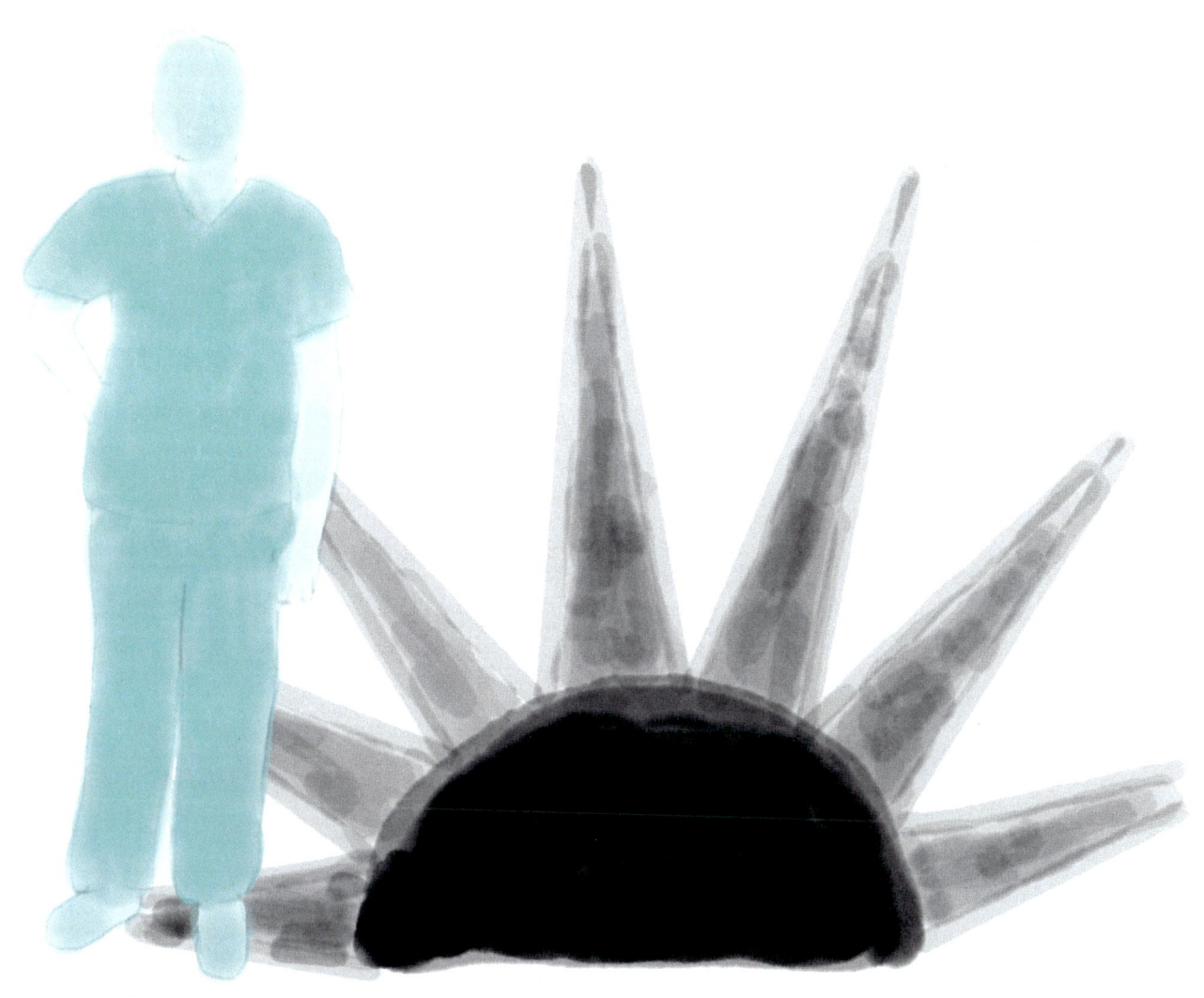

I love you in the early morning when your
night nurses say 'goodbye'.

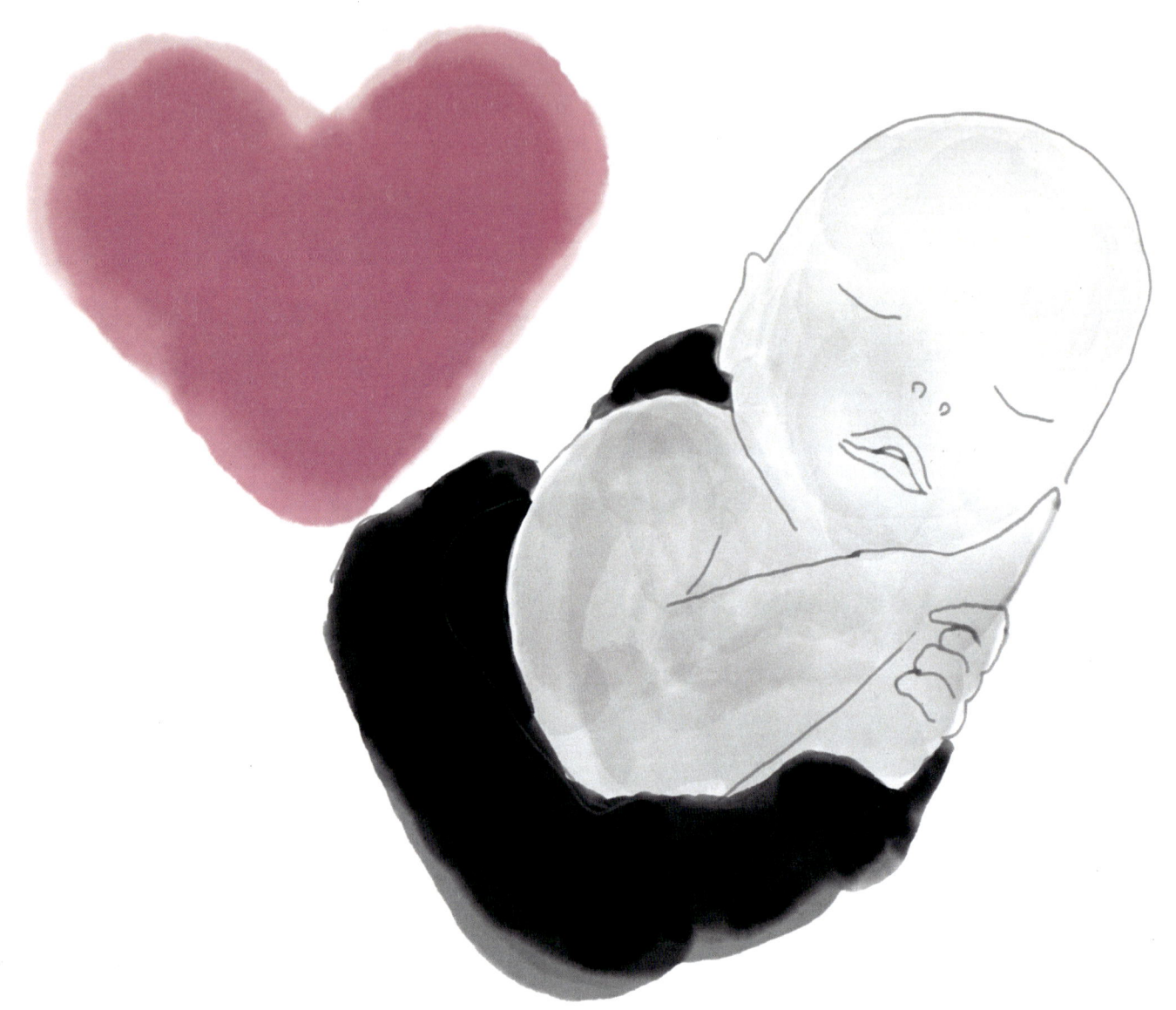

I love you in the long sleepy afternoons when
we lose track of what day and time it is.

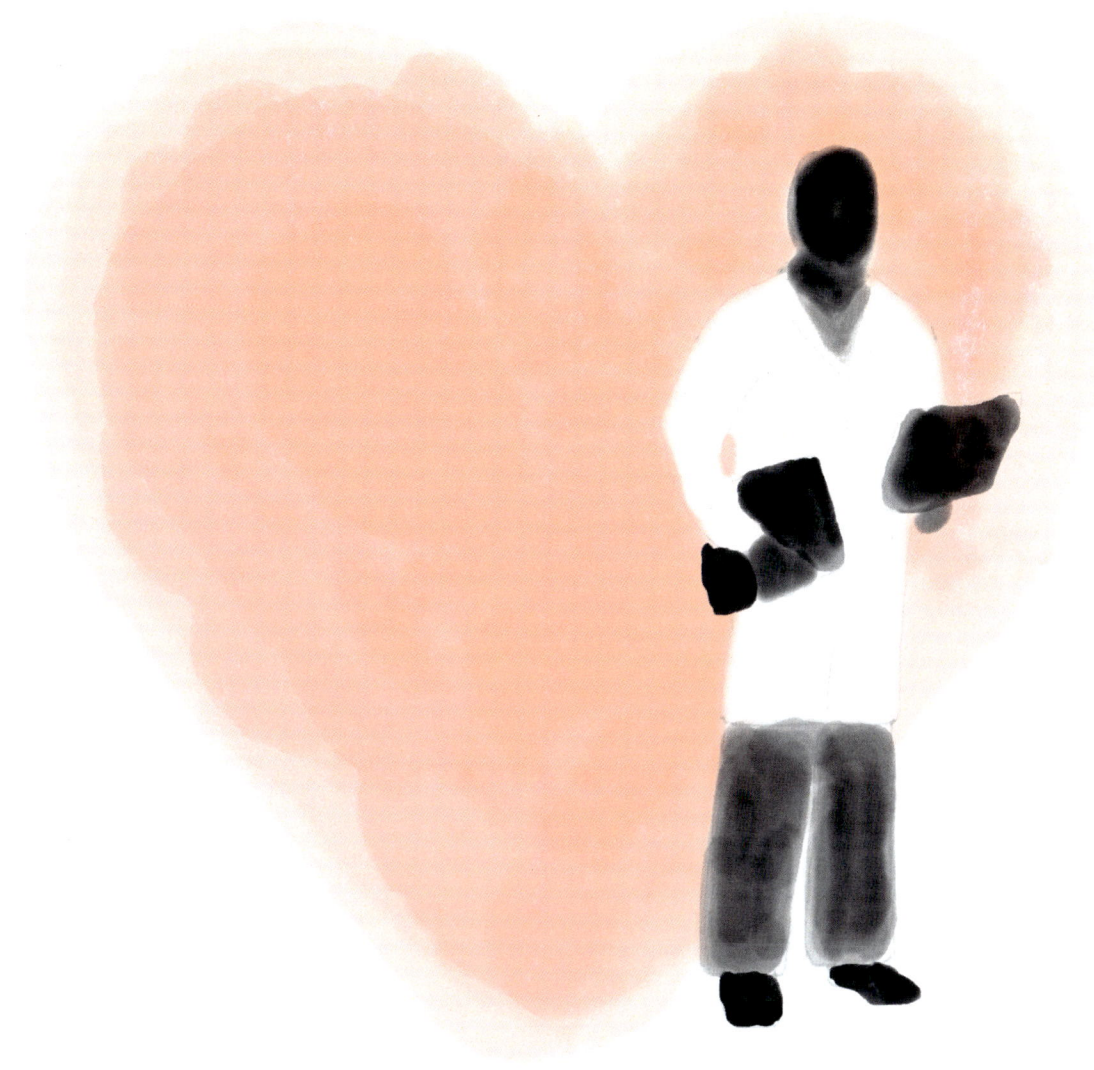

I love you when the doctors make their rounds, knowing all of your numbers and medicines.

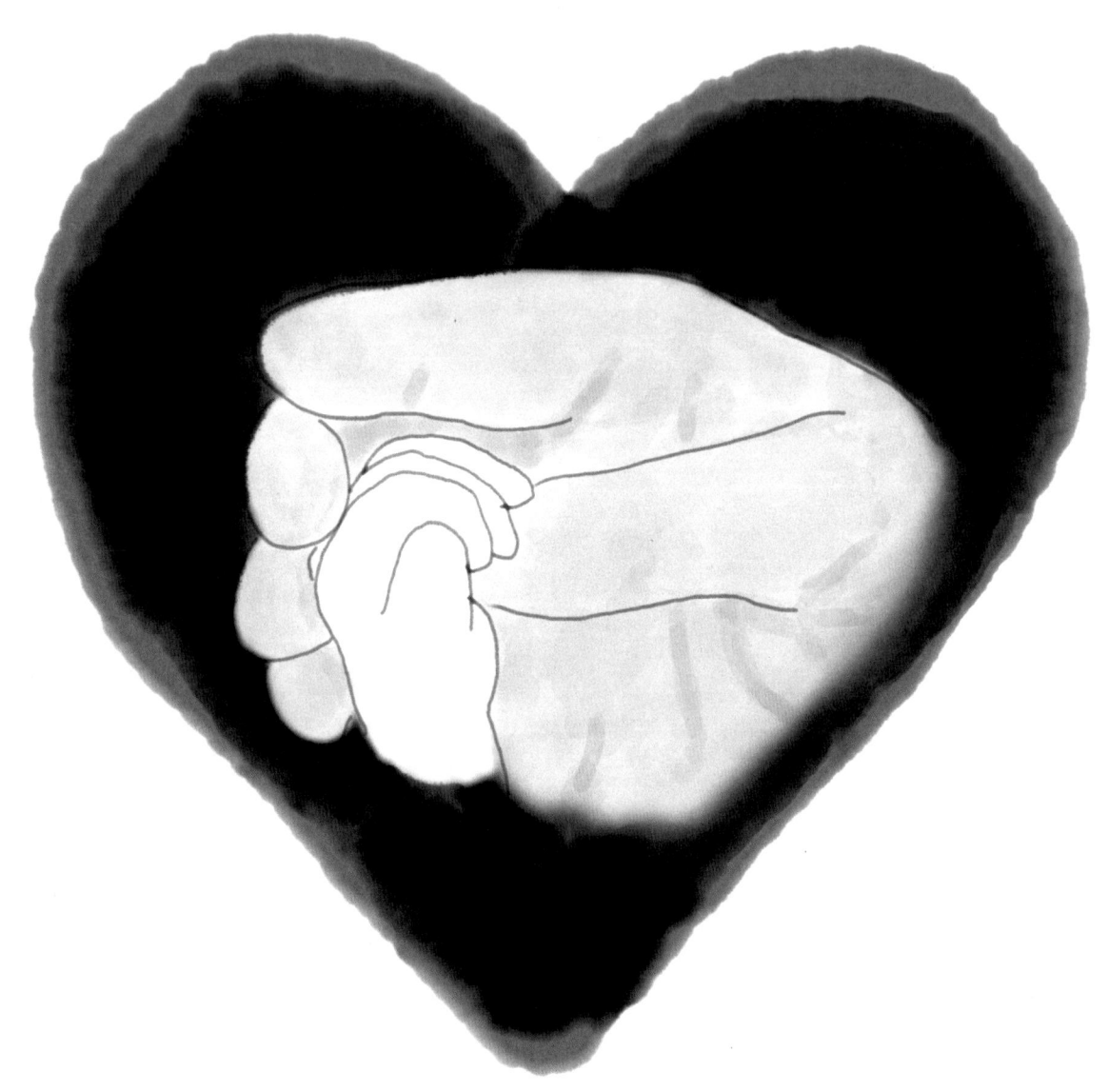

But, there are so many other things that
make you special.

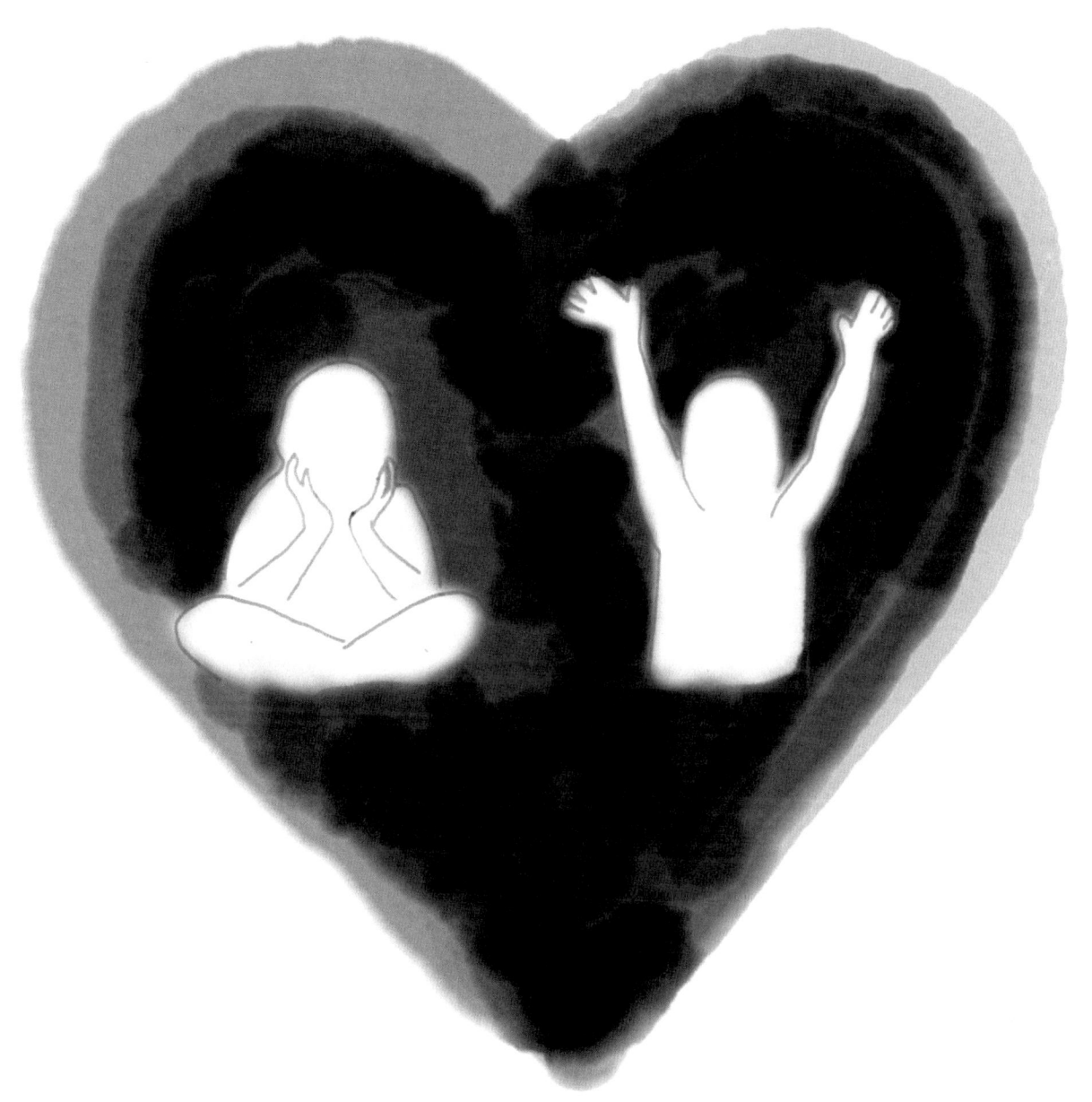

I love you on the hard days, and
I love you on the days filled with joy.

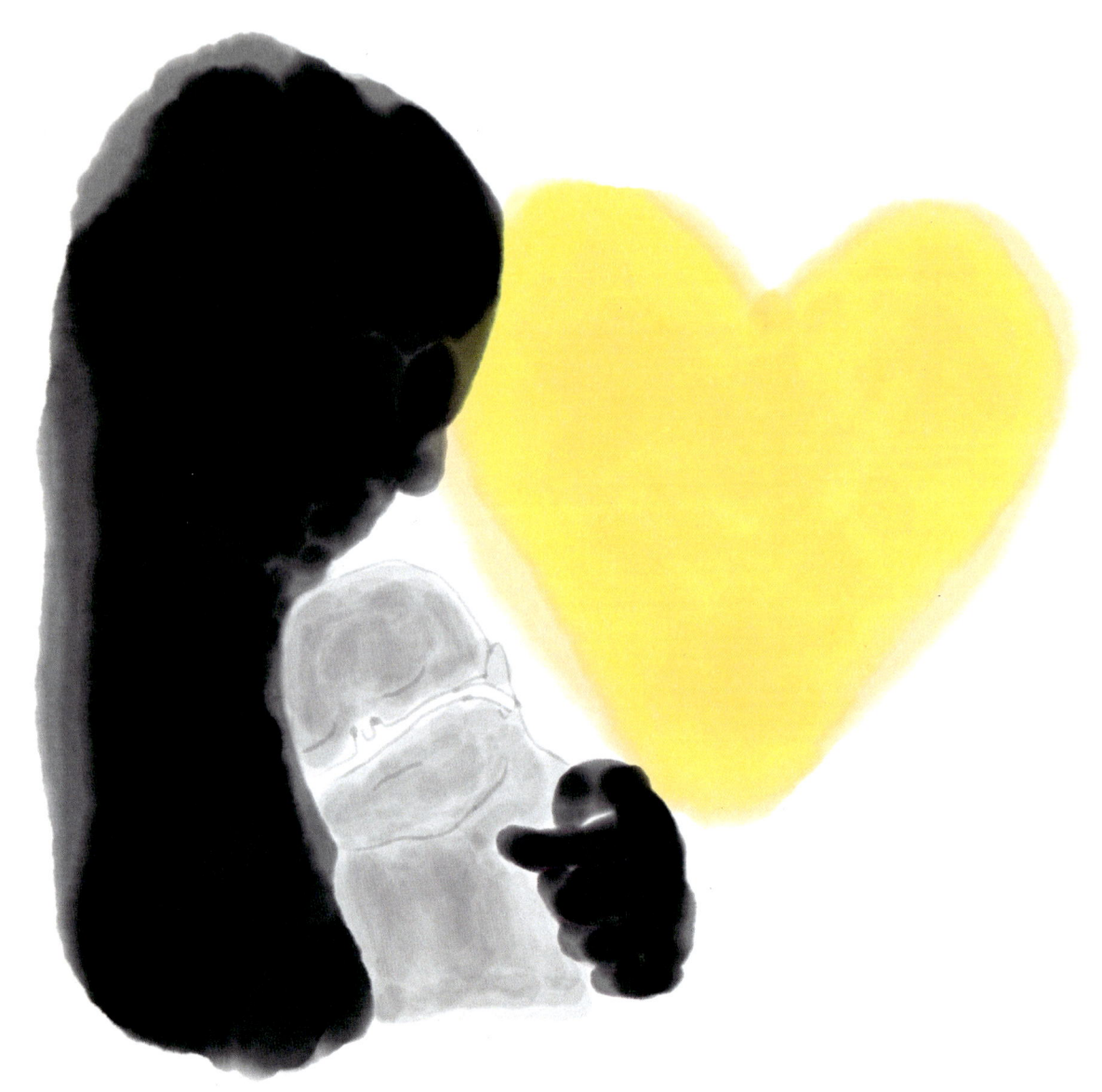

I love you when you do something new, and I love you when you take your time.

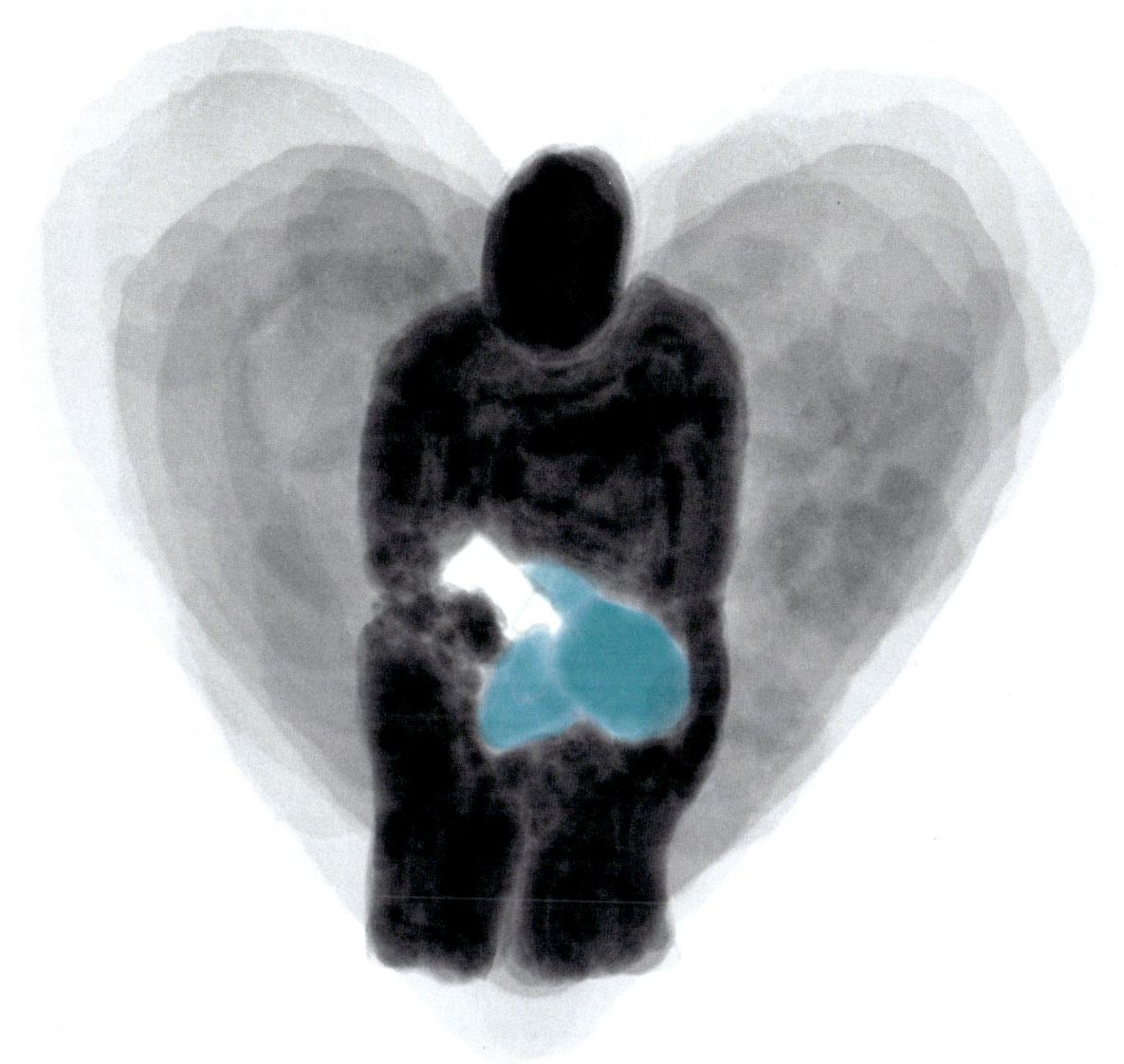

I love you when we get a step closer to going home, and I love you when we take a step back.

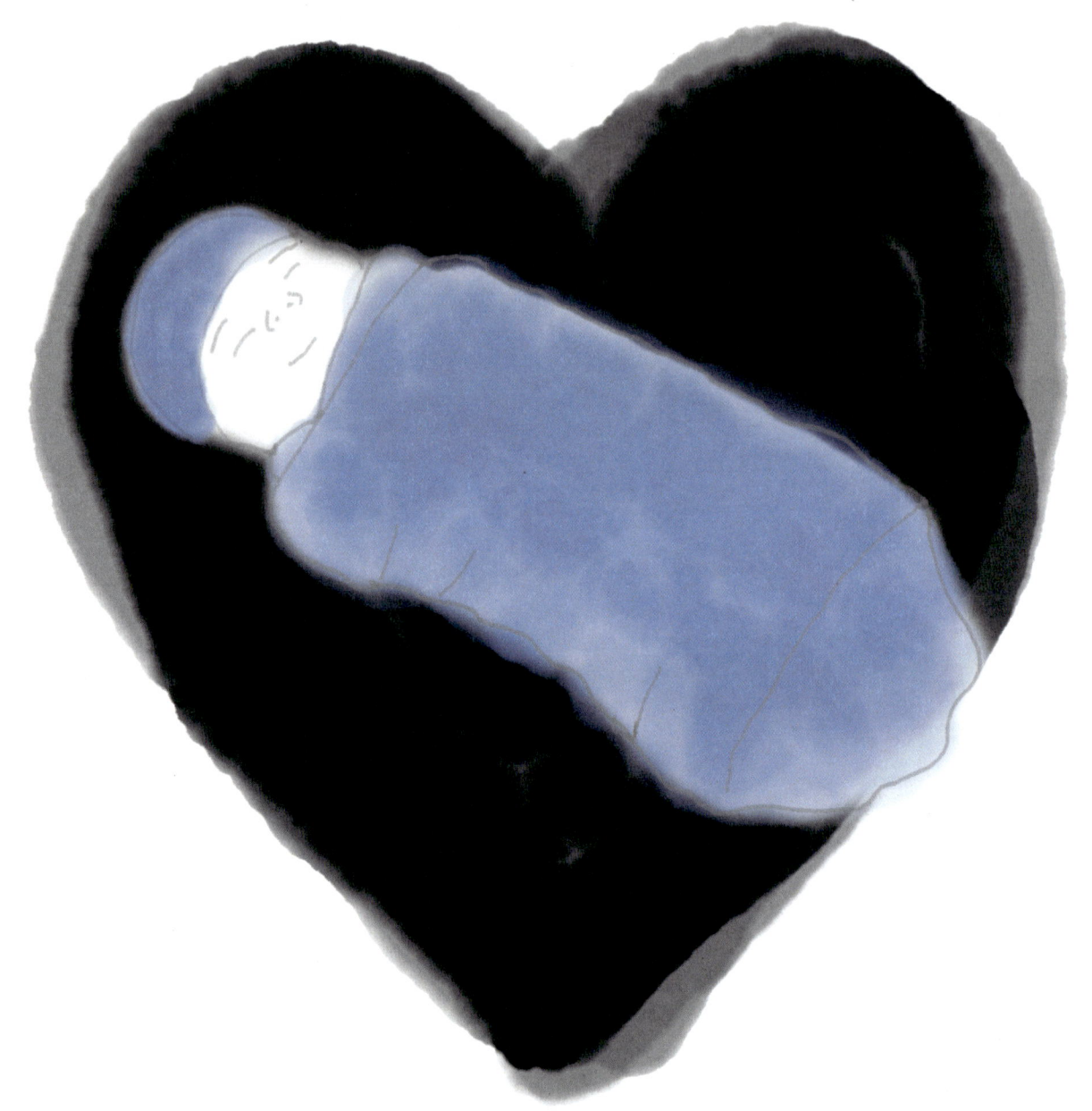

So, work hard little one. It will all be worth it.

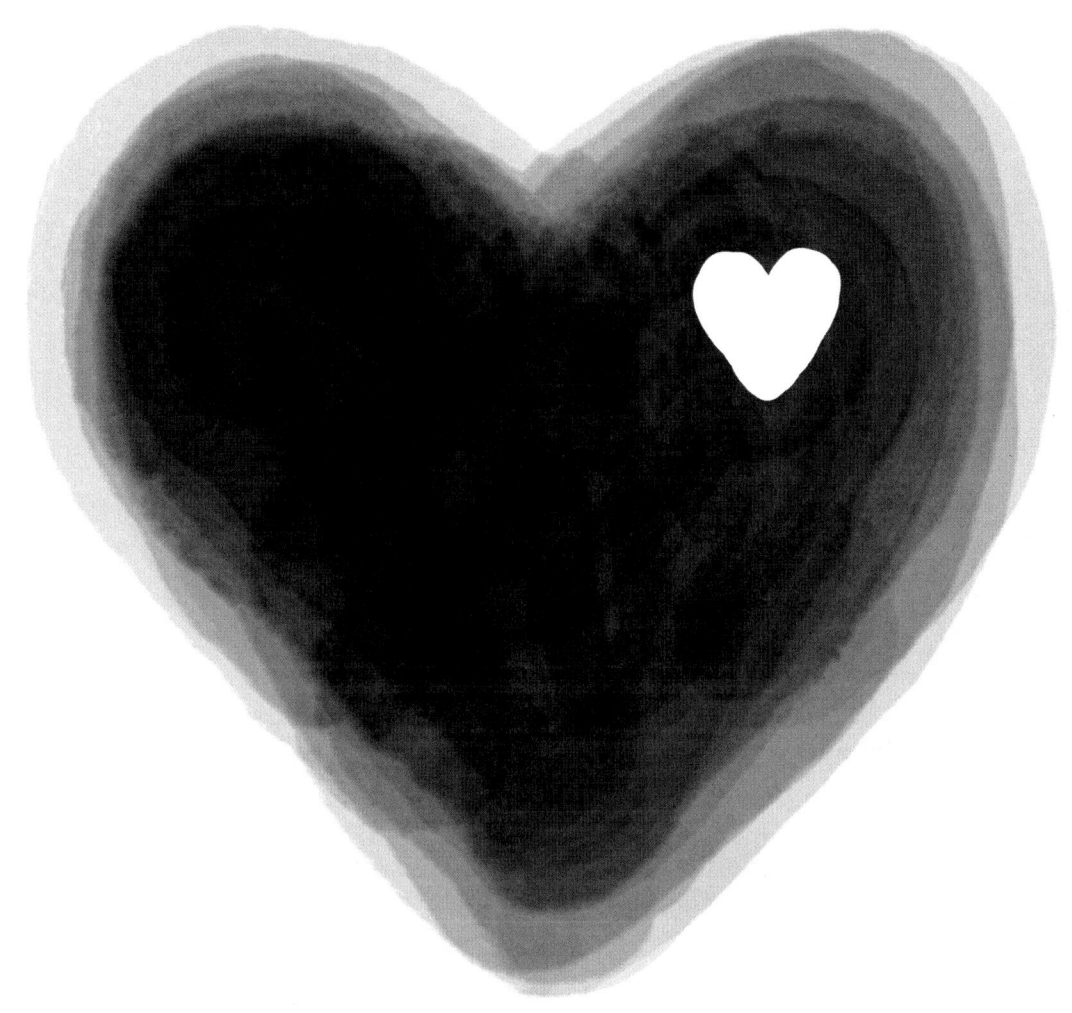

But, no matter where you are, what you do, and
how long we are here, I love you.

Laura Camerona, Certified Child Life Specialist

With a background in child development, Laura creates books that support children's needs and promote understanding. She specializes in writing books that help parents have hard conversations and support their children during hard times. She loves to partner with passionate people working in non-profit organizations to create books that support families dealing with a variety of struggles.

In a Laura's former career as a hospital Child Life Specialist, she worked in a variety of units, but her last 5 years were spent in the NICU. These families and staff hold a special place in her heart. Laura appreciates the many struggles that come hand and hand with a NICU stay. In this book, Laura focused on finding words that could support families in a large variety of circumstances and illustrations that were representative and inclusive.

Check out Laura's other books and services!

Instagram: @words.worth.repeating
Facebook: @WordsWorthRepeatingBooks
www.wordsworthrepeating.com

Will your baby be bringing home a new piece of medical equipment?

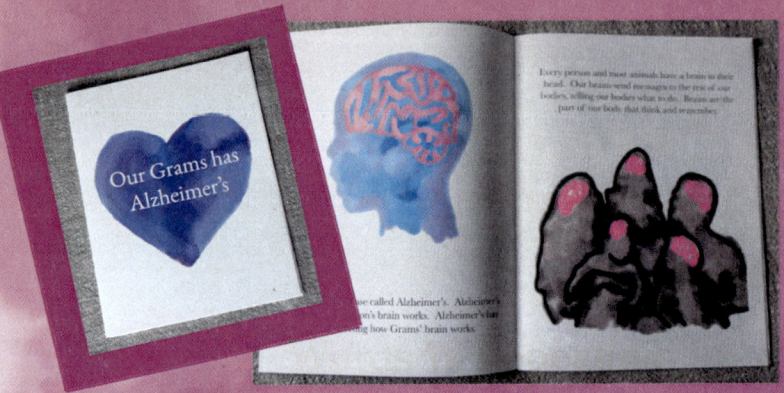

Words Worth Repeating creates books to promote positive coping and healing for kids and families.

Families work with a Child Life Specailist to create customized books that give famlies words for hard situations.

Has your baby received a new diagnosis and you are looking for ways to talk to your other kids about it?

Words Worth Repeating specializes in Journey Books (books about something a child or a loved one is experiencing) and Legacy Books (books about a loved one who has died).

Check out the website to learn more!

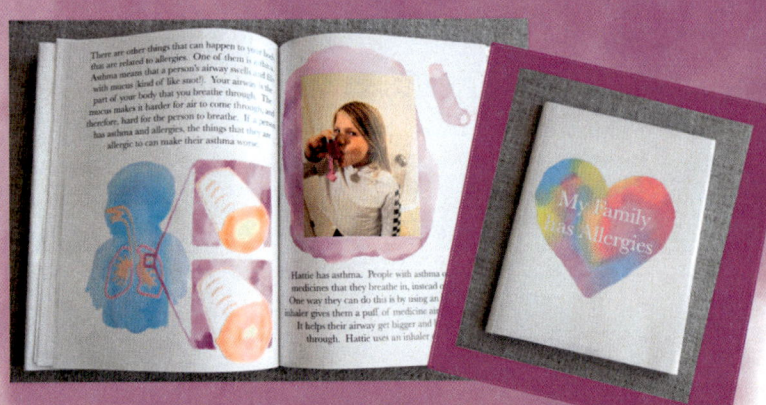

Let's make just the right book for your family!

Words Worth Repeating

www.wordsworthrepeating.com

Made in the USA
Monee, IL
30 December 2022